Henry Maunsell, Thomas More Madden

The Dublin Practice of Midwifery

Henry Maunsell, Thomas More Madden

The Dublin Practice of Midwifery

ISBN/EAN: 9783743420021

Manufactured in Europe, USA, Canada, Australia, Japa

Cover: Foto ©Andreas Hilbeck / pixelio.de

Manufactured and distributed by brebook publishing software (www.brebook.com)

Henry Maunsell, Thomas More Madden

The Dublin Practice of Midwifery

THE

DUBLIN PRACTICE

OF

MIDWIFERY.

BY

HENRY MAUNSELL, M.D.

FORMERLY PROFESSOR OF MIDWIFERY IN THE ROYAL COLLEGE
OF SURGEONS IN IRELAND;

ETC. ETC.

NEW EDITION, ENLARGED AND REVISED.

EDITED BY

THOMAS MORE MADDEN, M.R.I.A.

L.K.&Q.C.P.I., M.R.C.S. ENG., L.F.P. &c. GLASG.

Senior Assistant Physician, Rotunda, Dublin Lying-in Hospital;
Corresponding Member of the Gynæcological Society of Boston U.S.
Corresponding Fellow of the Edinburgh Obstetrical Society; &c.

LONDON:

LONGMANS, GREEN, AND CO.

1871.

EDITOR'S PREFACE.

———∘∘⦂⊗⦂∘∘———

A WORK which has passed through so many editions as Dr. Maunsell's 'Dublin Practice of Midwifery,' the practical value of which has been tested by the experience of thirty-six years, and which still remains the most popular compendium of the science it treats of, hardly requires any prefatory observations to introduce another edition. There are, however, some reasons which render this necessary on the present occasion.

In no department of medical science has such great practical progress taken place within the last few years as in the art of midwifery. The improvements which have been thus effected in obstetric science may be chiefly referred to four heads.

First. The more frequent and more timely use of the forceps in difficult labours, by which the mortality and sufferings of child-birth have been greatly diminished.

Secondly. The less frequent performance of craniotomy, and the substitution for it of other operations.

Thirdly. The treatment of post-partum hemorrhage by direct applications to the bleeding uterine vessels.

Fourthly. The treatment of puerperal fever, which has undergone a complete change of late years, owing in great measure to the alteration which has taken place in the prevailing type of disease.

As these changes have been effected by the progressive development of obstetric science since this work was first published, and as the author has for some time retired from active practice, much to the loss of this branch of medical science, it has been suggested to the present editor to revise and enlarge the work in these particulars, so as to make it a complete handbook of the present science and art of midwifery. This task he has undertaken with Dr. Maunsell's sanction.

The chief subjects in which alterations and additions have been made in this edition are the following :—The twelfth chapter, on the Use of the Forceps, has been completely re-written ; the fourteenth chapter, on the Treatment of Hemorrhage, has been considerably enlarged and altered. An additional chapter on the Present Type and Treatment of Puerperal Fever has been appended. The following chapters ' On the Third Order of Difficult Labours,' ' On Version in cases of Pelvic Deformity,' ' On the Cæsarean Section,' ' On the Induction of Premature Labour,' and that ' On Inversion of the Uterus,' are all entirely new.

The responsibility for these additions and changes, and for the opinions and statements advanced therein, rests entirely with the present editor. He may venture to observe that he has spared no pains to render this edition worthy of the high reputation which Dr. Maunsell's work has so long enjoyed, and of its position as a text-book of modern obstetric science. How far he has succeeded, it will be for the reader to judge.

ROTUNDA HOSPITAL, DUBLIN :
   January 1871.

PREFACE

THE FIRST EDITION.

———◆———

THOSE who are conversant with the teaching of obstetric medicine must have felt the difficulty of satisfactorily answering a question commonly put to them by students: What book do you recommend me to take to the Lying-in room? Yet there is, perhaps, no department of the healing art which can boast of more elaborate and valuable elementary systems than Midwifery. The works, however, of Denman and Burns, Ramsbotham and Merriman, though excellent in the Study, do not supply the want indicated in the question of the student. Their size and price (if there were nothing else) disqualify them for this service; and giving, as they do, the history

and principia of the science, conclusions and rules
cannot be obtained from them with the facility
and quickness desirable to the student and practitioner during the bustle of actual business.
In addition, as an Irish teacher of Midwifery, I
must say that though, in general principles, there
can be little room for disagreeing with the distinguished authors just named, still in many points
of practice the lessons of the Dublin school differ
materially from those inculcated in their books.
Of those publications upon the subject specially
intended as manuals, it does not become me to
speak ; and I shall, therefore, merely state shortly
what I have wished to do, and what to avoid, in
the construction of the present work.   My object,
then, has been to give a concise, but at the same
time sufficiently full and perfect account of practical Midwifery ; not merely to furnish an index
of hard-named diseases, and a jumbled catalogue
of discordant remedies, but to supply an available
knowledge of all appliances and means that are
known to be requisite for the safe conduct of a
patient through the perils and accidents of child-

birth. In attempting to attain this object, it has been my endeavour to state honestly my own practice, which, I believe, agrees pretty closely with that generally taught in the schools of this city, and upon important points will not be found to differ much from that recommended by the standard authorities in Midwifery. I have, however, given few or no references, as these can be easily obtained from the larger works, and here would have served merely to swell the book and dilute the matter, which it is desirable to offer in a form as concentrated as possible. In a word, remembering the strictures of Lord Bacon, it has been my wish, not so much to give 'a history large of bulk and pleasant for variety, but to weed out fables, quotations, needless controversies, and flourishes, which are more proper for table-talk and stories in a chimney-corner than for an institution in philosophy.' It is next to impossible to write a preface without egotism, and on that account a preface should be brief: this shall, therefore, be concluded by the simple statement that the material for the following pages was drawn exclusively from a syllabus of my lectures, without any works being at the time consulted upon the subject. By the adoption of this plan I hoped that the language and style might be found to possess a freshness not to be expected in a mere compilation. How far this and the other ends already alluded to may have been attained, must now be left to the judgment of the profession.

York Street, Dublin:
August 1834.

CONTENTS.

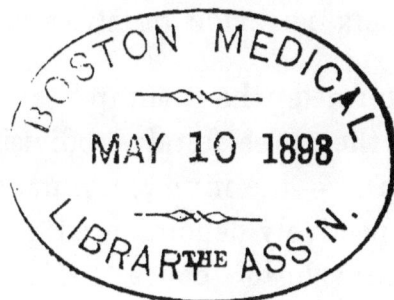

DUBLIN PRACTICE

OF

MIDWIFERY.

CHAPTER I.

THE PELVIS.

IT IS CUSTOMARY to commence the study of Midwifery with the consideration of the bony structure of the pelvis; a knowledge of the anatomy of this part being, in fact, essentially requisite for the understanding of the mechanism whereby the fœtus is, either naturally or artificially, transmitted into the world. At present I shall strictly confine my observations to such of its properties as may be of obstetric interest, other points being sufficiently noticed in surgical and anatomical works.

The pelvis, then, is a firm osseous case, formed in the adult of four bones—the two ossa innominata, sacrum, and coccyx. The two latter are

B

popularly termed the 'rump' and 'huckle'
bones; and the three fœtal subdivisions of each
os innominatum—the ilium, ischium, and pubis—
are also respectively denominated the 'haunch,'
'sitting,' and 'shear' bones. A knowledge of
these vernacular names will often enable us to
comprehend more clearly the descriptions of
patients, especially those in the lower classes of
society.

These different bones are connected to one
another by four articulations.

Two serve to unite the sacrum with the os innominatum of either side. These are denominated
the sacro-iliac synchondroses, and possess remarkable strength, both from the manner in which the
prominences and hollows of the opposed surfaces
are, as it were, morticed into each other, and also
from the strong bands of ligament stretched across
the posterior and upper edges. A ligamentous
expansion further strengthens the front of the
articulation; but this is thin and membranous,
that it may not, by its bulk, diminish the capacity
of the pelvic cavity. Two other remarkable ligaments on either side connect the sacrum and ossa
innominata, but seem rather intended to complete
the walls of the pelvis than to add security to the
joint. These are the anterior and posterior sacro-
sciatic ligaments, both arising from the sides of the
sacrum and coccyx, and attached, the former to

the spine, and the latter to the tuberosity of the ischium.

The third pelvic articulation is that between the two ossa innominata themselves, and denominated the *symphysis pubis*. This differs from the sacro-iliac synchondroses in having an interarticular substance interposed between the two osseous surfaces, in addition to the fibro-cartilage covering each of these. The joint is secured by bands of ligament, which, for the reason already assigned, are stronger and more bulky externally. There is also a ligament termed the sub-pubic, which occupies the apex of the arch formed by the rami of the pubic bones.

The last articulation is that between the sacrum and coccyx. In it the union is effected by an interposed substance analogous to that between the vertebræ, and is secured by ligaments anteriorly and posteriorly. The sacro-coccygeal joint is capable of flexion and extension to a considerable extent, and is the only one in the pelvis naturally admitting of motion. In certain animals, as the cow, the other articulations become relaxed about the period of parturition ; and it has been surmised by some authors, but without sufficient proof, that a similar relaxation always occurs in the human female.

The pelvis, formed, as we have described, of several bones firmly united together, has been, by one of those whimsical resemblances of which anatomists are so fond, declared to be conical in shape. Little information, however, is to be acquired from this description; and a much better idea of the properties of the pelvis will be conveyed by stating its average or standard measurements, which the student can verify by examining the bones for himself.

Before proceeding to this statement, we must observe that the entire *case* is divided into two portions by the bony ridge or angle which, dividing the body from the ala of the os innominatum, is denominated the ileo-pectineal line. The space above this line is termed the hypogastric cavity, or false pelvis; that below it the true, or lesser pelvis. The hypogastric cavity possesses no bony wall anteriorly, but is bounded laterally and posteriorly by the alæ of the ilii and the lumbar vertebræ. Its dimensions vary much, and are of minor importance to the obstetric student; but the distance from the top of one ilium to the other, at the widest, is, in a standard pelvis, between ten and eleven inches; and that between the two antero-superior spinous processes somewhat more than nine inches.

We now come to the consideration of the true or lesser pelvis, which, from its forming the unyielding boundary of the canal through which the mature fœtus is to be transmitted, is more closely allied to our present subject. In describing and measuring this canal, three portions are usually specified : the brim, called also the superior strait or introitus ; the 'cavity ; and the outlet, or inferior strait or detroitus.

The *brim* formed by the ileo-pectineal lines and the angle of union between the sacrum and lumbar vertebræ is somewhat elliptical in shape, the regularity of the figure being interrupted behind by the projection of the promontory or base of the sacrum. The dimensions of this aperture are measured by four lines passing through its centre: the longest of these, passing from side to side, and denominated the transverse diameter, is usually about five inches and a quarter in length ; the shortest, being that drawn from the centre of the base of the sacrum to the symphysis pubis, and termed the antero-posterior, or conjugate diameter, measures in the standard female pelvis four inches and a quarter. The two remaining lines, called the oblique diameters, are those stretching from the sacro-iliac articulation on one side, to the back of the acetabulum on the other. The length of each of these is commonly five inches. By many authors the last diameter is mentioned as the longest—a mistake arising from the circumstance of its actually being so in the *recent* pelvis; the length of the transverse diameter being then somewhat diminished by the prominence of the psoæ muscles and great vessels and nerves.

The *outlet*, or inferior aperture, presents in the dry preparation an extremely irregular figure, its margin being interrupted by three deep triangular notches ; viz. the two sciatic, and that between the rami of the pubes. In the recent subject, however, the two former are subtended by the sacro-sciatic ligaments, in such a manner as to give the aperture a quadrilateral character. Its dimensions are described by two lines: one, passing between the inner margins of the tubera ischii, and called the transverse diameter, averages in length four inches; the other, denominated the long, or antero-posterior diameter, is stretched between the inferior margin of the symphysis pubis and the tip of the sacrum, and measures five inches. In examining a pelvis, with the coccyx attached, it will be observed that the distance between the same point of the symphysis and the tip of this bone is not more than four inches. Owing, however, to the mobility of the sacro-coccygeal joint, the space admits of being enlarged to five inches, or to the full extent of the distance between the point of the sacrum and the lower margin of the symphysis. In making these measurements it is also to be noted, that the directions of the long and short diameters of the brim and outlet are reversed—a provision of which a beautiful and satisfactory explanation will appear, when we come to examine the relative dimensions of the mature fœtus.

While considering the outlet of the pelvis, we may conveniently notice the arch of the pubis. This is much wider, and assumes more the form of an arch in the female than in the male; in the former also its rami are bevelled in such a manner as to give a direction forwards to any body passing through the canal of the pelvis. A line subtending this arch measures about three inches.

The cavity of the pelvis, being more capacious than either the brim or outlet, does not require to be accurately measured; nor, from its peculiar form, would it be easy to measure it. We may remark, however, how admirably the hollow of the sacrum (for this purpose deeper in the female than in the male) is adapted for the lodgment of the bulky face of the child, while the convergence of the point of the sacrum and spines of the ischia is well calculated to second the bevelling of the rami pubis in directing the vertex forwards. The depth of the female pelvis now remains to be ascertained, and we shall find it to differ much in different parts. At the symphysis pubis it is seldom more than one inch and a half. At the sides, from the brim to the tubera ischii it is about three inches and a half, and behind, a right line drawn from the base to the tip of the sacrum measures, generally, four and a half or five inches. From this irregularity of depth in different parts, we may easily see, that a body may be close to the outlet anteriorly, while it still has to traverse a considerable length of the back and sides of the passage.

The bearing of the pelvis on the trunk claims some attention. In the erect posture of the body, the axis of the trunk being perpendicular, there would have been constant danger of prolapsus of the viscera, if the axis of the pelvic passage had been continuous with it. This, however, is not the case; but the line representing the latter axis bisects the axis of the trunk so obliquely as to form an angle inferiorly of about thirty-five degrees. In other words, were the axis of the trunk produced downwards, it would fall, not upon the centre of the pelvic aperture, but upon the symphysis pubis.

In the foregoing observations, we have, to avoid confusion, spoken of the axis of the pelvis in the ordinary sense of that term, as if it were a right line passing through the centre of the passage. No such *right* line, however, can exist; for the whole pelvis is so bent that both its brim and outlet look toward the forepart of the body; and the axis of the former, or a right line passing through its centre, would, if produced downwards, fall upon the point of the sacrum: while the axis of the outlet, if produced upwards, would strike the promontory of that bone. Hence it is obvious, that what obstetricians mean by the axis of the pelvis must be a *curved* line, passing respectively through the centres of both brim and outlet, and nearly corresponding in its curvature to that of the sacrum. The practical deductions from these facts are, that a body to get into the pelvis through the brim must pass downwards, and *backwards*; and to get out of it, at the outlet, must proceed downwards and *forwards*.

The foregoing are the chief points of obstetric interest in a standard female pelvis. Deviations are occasionally met with, and may consist either in deformity of shape; in deficiency, or in excess of capacity.

The most usual cause of deformity of the pelvis is, doubtless, the occurrence of *rickets* during infancy, when the bones, not being possessed of sufficient firmness, are pressed from their natural positions by the weight of the trunk and counteracting resistance of the lower extremities. The same effect is said to be produced, in a similar way, by the disease called *mollities ossium*; and deformity may also, sometimes, be occasioned by fractures, or the occurrence of exostosis. The contraction of the passage from rickets generally occurs at the brim, and oftener from before backward than in the lateral direction. It, however, may exist in a great variety of forms, and occasionally is so extreme that the canal is compressed into a T-shaped slit. In some cases the capacity of the aperture will be much diminished at one side, while, at the other, little or no alteration will be observable. It is said, that in many cases the deformity will actually increase after every successive labour, and that the act of parturition, which was, perhaps, at first only difficult, may, after some repetitions, become absolutely impossible without artificial aid.

The pelvis, without being deformed, is in some instances unusually small, and should the foetus then happen to be disproportionately large, it is obvious that the same effects must be produced, as if the passage was *morbidly* diminished in size. On the other hand, we have said, that the pelvis may deviate from the standard in having an excessive capacity, in which case the attendant inconveniences will be, liability to retroversion and prolapsus of the uterus, and to sudden unexpected delivery.

The dimensions, and other characters just mentioned, can all be easily enough ascertained upon the dry bones, but when we come to enquire into them in the living body, we find it quite another affair. With the view of assisting the enquiry, several instruments have been invented, the most remarkable of which are—the pelvimeter of Coutouli, and the callipers of Baudelocque. The latter were to be used externally, to measure the size of the pelvis, in a way precisely similar to that in which they are employed by mechanics. The former resembled a shoemaker's rule, one limb of which was to be thrust into the vagina, and planted against the promontory of the sacrum, while the other, moving upon a graduated rod, was to be brought into contact with the symphysis pubis, thus pointing out the measurement of the antero-posterior diameter. It is unnecessary to do more than mention those fantastic contrivances, their inefficiency and inapplicability being fully recognised by British accoucheurs.

We can, however, generally obtain useful information by the employment of the fingers alone, and a few remarks on the mode of using them will be necessary. By passing the index finger into the vagina, and carrying it upwards and backwards, we can in many cases touch the promontory of the sacrum, and if we then mark the part of the finger or edge of the hand in contact with the arch of the pubis, we can easily, by making a trifling deduction for the thickness of the symphysis and the obliquity of the finger's direction, estimate the length of the conjugate diameter. But sometimes, while this diameter is of sufficient extent, considerable contraction may exist on one or both sides of it. In such a case, a sharp angle must be formed at the back of the symphysis, and on this point we can satisfy ourselves by introducing two or three fingers into the vagina, and placing them in contact with the part; if they lie evenly, side by side, there can be no very acute angle, and consequently no remarkable diminution of capacity on their side of the conjugate diameter. By using the fingers, we are also enabled to discover any irregular ridges of bone, or tumours, that may have the effect of diminishing the capacity of the passage.

CHAPTER II.

THE FŒTUS.

WE MAY NOW advantageously turn our attention
to the properties of the fœtus, so far as they relate to its passage through the pelvic canal.

While in the womb, the various parts of the
child are packed together in such a manner as to
occupy the least possible space, forming a mass
somewhat of an oval shape. The head is flexed, so
as to bring the chin upon the thorax, the arms
are applied to the sides, and the forearms and
hands flexed and applied, often crossing each
other, to the breast; the thighs are flexed on the
abdomen, and the legs upon the thighs, the feet
often, like the hands, crossing each other. In this
way the head forms one extremity of the oval we
have mentioned, while the other is composed of
the feet and nates.

The fœtus, we are to observe, is somewhat
flexible in a lateral direction, very much so anteriorly, and but little posteriorly. The parts of it

requiring to be particularly measured and examined are the head, the shoulders, and the
breech. The first more especially demands our
attention, both as being, upon the whole, most
bulky and least compressible, and also as being
the part which is usually first engaged in the
pelvic passages.

The head of the fœtus, detached and without
the face, is described as oval, with the large extremity posteriorly. The desire of pointing out
resemblances seems to be a besetting passion with
anatomists; but in truth, in this, as in many other
instances, the likening of the head to any known
figure conveys but little information. The student,
then, who desires correct notions upon the subject,
must set before him a fœtal skull of the standard
(or average) dimensions and shape, and carefully
examine upon it the properties which I shall now
endeavour to indicate.

The first circumstance that strikes us in our
examination is the great mobility of the bones
upon each other, owing to their incomplete ossification and the cartilaginous connection between
them. This effect is also increased by the prolongation of the sagittal suture through the centre of
the os frontis, so as actually to divide it into two
bones, and it can be produced to such an extent
as to admit of the bulk of the head being considerably diminished in one of its diameters, and

proportionally increased in another. The situation and yielding nature of the sutures require to be attended to; their general direction is the same as in the adult, but the sagittal is always prolonged, as we have mentioned, to the root of the nose : sometimes, but rarely, it passes backward into the occipital bone. At the junction of the lambdoid and sagittal sutures, owing to the non-ossification of the occipital and parietal bones, a triangular space is left, closed only by cartilage, and called the lesser or posterior fontanelle. A similar but larger space occurs between the parietal and frontal bones, at the intersection of the coronal and sagittal sutures. This is termed the greater or anterior fontanelle, and is distinguishable by being lozenge-shaped, and having four concurrent sutures, while the former is triangular, and has only three concurrent sutures. A knowledge of the differences between these fontanelles may sometimes assist us in a diagnosis of the situation of the head during labour.

We shall now enquire into the dimensions of the standard fœtal head, which are usually measured by lines, somewhat loosely denominated diameters.

The shortest of these is the bi-parietal, or that stretched between the tuberosities of the parietal bones on either side, and is about three inches and a half, or three inches and a quarter in length;

this, it is plain, can meet with no obstruction in passing through any part of the *standard* pelvis, the shortest diameter of the latter being nowhere less than four inches.

There are, however, three other measurements to be considered, which, from being all in the long axis of the head, are usually called the long diameters. One or other of these, together with the bi-parietal diameter, may be considered as the measure of the bulk of the passing body, in every head presentation.

The shortest, and that which is most usually opposed to the long diameters of the pelvis, is described by an imaginary right line, extending from the upper part of the forehead to the lower part of the occiput. This can only become the opposing diameter when the chin is very much depressed toward the chest, as it usually is, the vertex being the presenting part. The length of this line is about four inches, which, it will be remembered, is not greater than the shortest diameter of the pelvis, but as it is naturally opposed to the longest diameters of that passage, there can, of course, be no want of room in such a case. Such, then, are the relations, as to dimensions, between the head and pelvis under the most favourable circumstances.

The next in length of the great diameters, is that between the lower part of the forehead and the upper part of the occiput. It usually measures four inches and a half, being about half an inch longer than the last. This comes to be the opposing diameter in that variety of head presentation in which the head is extended upon the neck and the forehead applied towards the pubis, called also the fontanelle presentation, in consequence of the anterior fontanelle being in such cases the presenting part.

The longest diameter of the head is that between the point of the chin and the vertex. It measures five inches, and is the opposing diameter in another variety of natural presentation, viz. when the face is the presenting part: it must be obvious that this position of the head will materially increase the difficulties of its transit.

The *depth* of the head, from the sagittal suture to the occipital foramen, may be estimated at about three inches and a quarter.

The dimensions, of course, vary in different individuals, but those we have given are about the average. The heads of female children are usually somewhat less than those of males; Dr. Joseph Clarke* estimates the difference at one-twenty-eighth or one-thirtieth of the circumference.

The movements of the head now claim a little attention. These are, flexion forwards and extension backwards, both, especially the former,

* Phil. Trans. v. 76.

capable of being carried to a considerable extent. Direct lateral inclination is only admitted to a slight degree, and rotation can be carried just so far as to allow of the chin resting on the shoulder, but not farther without endangering the child's safety.

We have spoken of variations from the natural form and average size of the pelvic passage, and we shall also be able to detect similar deviations from the standard in the head of the fœtus. It may, for instance, be very small, which of course will have no effect, except to facilitate its expulsion. It may, on the other hand, be very large, and if it be so, disproportionately with the size of the pelvis, difficult labour will be the consequence, and it is even possible that the use of instruments may be necessary. On this point, however, it is proper to think with caution, as the extraordinary change of shape which may be effected on the head by compression will often suffice to counterbalance even a considerable disproportion of size.

The head is occasionally enlarged, while in the womb, by hydrocephalus, and may require diminution by means of instruments: the head of a dead fœtus is also sometimes swollen by the air disengaged during putrefaction. A peculiar form of head is not *very* rarely met with, in which the upper portion of the cranium is malformed, and partly deficient, and the place of the brain occupied by a sort of fungous mass. These are denominated acephalous, or (by the Germans) cat-headed fœtuses : they may create confusion in our first examinations by wanting the peculiar firm feel of the natural head, but they are not often productive of difficulty in the act of parturition.

The shoulders of the fœtus are generally about five inches in breadth, but the effect of their size is counteracted by their possessing capability of motion to such an extent, that one can precede the other in their entry into the pelvis.

From what has been said, it is obvious that the long axes of the head and shoulders decussate, or are at right angles with each other ; and we can now perceive the value of a similar arrangement which we adverted to before, of the long diameters of the brim and outlet of the pelvis. At the moment when the head is escaping in the most favourable manner through the latter, the shoulders are accommodated in the long diameter of the former.

We have next to say a word upon the pelvic extremity of the fœtus, as it is packed in the uterus, and sometimes presents in the pelvic passage. Occasionally, the nates form the whole bulk of the presenting part; at other times the feet present along with them ; and again, the feet or knees pass first into the world. These differences make a good deal of variation in the antero-posterior diameter of the pelvic extremity, but it is almost always less than the transverse, which pretty constantly measures four inches.

Presentation and position.—Before proceeding to the consideration of the mode in which the child is propelled through the pelvis, or, as it is called, the mechanism of parturition, we shall briefly explain the meaning we attach to two words which we shall frequently employ, and which, indeed, have been already made use of in the preceding observations.   The words alluded to are, *presentation,* and *position.*   By the first we wish to designate that part of the child which, during labour, may be opposite the centre of the pelvic passage : and by the second, the relative position of the child with respect to the bones of the mother's pelvis.   Thus, if we say the vertex presents, we announce the presentation ; and if we add, with the occiput toward the pubis, or toward the sacrum, as the case may be, we describe the position.

CHAPTER III.

MECHANISM OF PARTURITION.

WE HAVE NOW to consider the modes in which nature essays to accomplish the transit of the mature fœtus through the bony canal of the pelvis, and we shall find, that of these there are three grand varieties; viz. presentations of the head; of the breech or lower limbs; and of the upper limbs, or side of the body.

In either of the two first varieties the fœtus presents an extremity of its long axis, and a brief consideration of the various measurements and characters described in the last chapter, will be sufficient to explain, that in ordinary cases no material obstacle to its passage can exist. In the third variety, the side of the child presenting, the long axis lies transversely to the pelvic aperture, and can only be expelled under peculiar circumstances (afterwards to be explained), to the production of which nature unassisted is rarely competent.

In a great majority of cases the head is the presenting part; and we shall, therefore, first examine the mechanism of its transmission.

Some varieties occur as to the *position* in which the head enters the brim of the pelvis; and of these, French authors have, with their usual ingenuity, taken advantage, and confused the subject by at least seven subdivisions. For practical purposes, however, such minuteness is unnecessary, and satisfactory notions upon the subject may be conveyed by explanations of three varieties. In the first and most common, the head enters the brim of the pelvis with the sagittal suture in the direction of either of its oblique diameters, and the posterior fontanelle applied to the back of either *acetabulum*. In the second, the sagittal suture is still in the same direction, but the posterior fontanelle is applied to either sacro-iliac *synchondrosis*. In this variety the head occasionally, but rarely, is expelled with the face toward the pubis. In the third variety the face is the presenting part.

In the *first position*, then, the head enters the brim of the pelvis with its posterior fontanelle directed toward either acetabulum (generally to the left), and the forehead directed toward either sacro-iliac synchondrosis (generally to the right). The presenting part, or that which we may touch most readily upon introducing a finger into the outlet of the pelvis, is the superior portion of one of the parietal bones near its tuber ; consequently, the head descends obliquely into the pelvis, neither the vertex nor the sagittal suture being the lowest part, but one of the parietal bones; the right, when the posterior fontanelle is directed toward the left acetabulum, and the left when it lies toward the opposite side. By this oblique position of the head, its transverse diameter is rendered somewhat less than that which would be described by a line passing between the two parietal tuberosities, which, if the vertex was the lowest or presenting part, would be the moving transverse diameter. During this stage of the process, the chin of the fœtus is depressed upon its chest, so as to bring the shortest of the long diameters of the head, or that between the lower part of the occiput and the upper part of the forehead, into the direction of the oblique or longest diameter of the mother's pelvis. At this time the greater fontanelle or the vertex is lower than the lesser, and being situated anteriorly, can, from the shallowness of that portion of the pelvis, be felt very near the external opening. As the head descends, the face turns somewhat into the hollow of the sacrum, and the vertex approaches the symphysis pubis. It is, however, the parietal bone which first escapes, and the vertex does not reach the anterior central line until in the very act of being expelled from the outlet. The mechanism by which this *turning* is accomplished is extremely interesting. The hollow of the sacrum is provided for the reception of the bulky face of the child, while the convergence of the point of the sacrum and spines of the ischia, and the bevelling of the inner surfaces of the rami pubis, form so many inclined planes, upon which the round smooth cranium is guided forward under the pubic arch. The change effected at the expulsion of the head brings, at the same instant, the long diameter of the shoulders obliquely into the brim of the pelvis, thus taking advantage of the wise adaptation (already alluded to), by which the long diameters of the brim and outlet are placed at right angles with each other. The head, soon after its expulsion, is again turned with the face toward one thigh of the mother, and thereby the greatest breadth of the shoulders from side to side is brought into the direction of the long diameter of the outlet from before backwards: the rest of the body and limbs follow without difficulty.

Second position of the head.—In this, which is of much less frequent occurrence than the first position, the posterior fontanelle is directed toward either sacro-iliac synchondrosis (generally to the right), and the forehead directed toward either acetabulum (generally to the left). The presenting part is the upper and fore part of one of the parietal bones, the head, as in the first position, descending obliquely into the pelvis. As the force of the uterus continues to act upon the head, the round and bulky vertex and tuberosity of one parietal bone are directed against the inclined plane formed by one of the spines of the ischia, and by it guided forwards toward the neighbouring acetabulum, while the less bulky but smooth forehead is, by the same motion, passed backwards toward the sacro-iliac synchondrosis of its own side. In this situation the head is expelled, the case being, in fact, converted into one of the first position. This, I believe, is the usual course; Professor Nägele of Heidelberg observed it to occur in ninety-three out of ninety-six cases.

In some few instances, however, the vertex, instead of being directed forwards, as has been described above, is turned toward the sacrum, and the upper and fore part of one of the parietals passes out first under the arch of the pubis, constituting a presentation with the *face to the pubis*. This is a less favourable position than the first, as the head passes, not flexed, but extended upon the trunk; and, consequently, the moving diameter is the second in length, being that between the lower part of the forehead and the upper part of the occiput. It is said by some, that the head occasionally presents at the brim with the forehead directly toward the pubis, and the vertex directly backwards, but this, I believe, never occurs, except in the case of a very small head.

Third position, or face presentation.—In this variety the face usually enters the brim of the pelvis with the forehead toward one sacro-iliac synchondrosis (generally the left), and the chin toward the opposite acetabulum (generally the right). The presenting part, then, is the upper portion of one cheek. As the labour advances, the chin is directed under the pubic arch, and passes first out of the pelvis. Occasionally, but rarely, the forehead will be, at the commencement, directed forwards toward one of the acetabula, and the chin may turn back toward the hollow of the sacrum. In one case, however, in which I distinctly ascertained this to be the situation at the commencement, the chin was subsequently turned forwards in the manner described above as happening in the second position, and was expelled first under the pubis. In face presentations, the moving diameter of the head is its longest, being that between the chin and vertex.

Presentations of the nates and lower extremities.—When the child is transmitted through the pelvis with its nates or lower limbs foremost, its position admits of two varieties. The first and most frequent, is with the back of the child inclined toward the abdomen of the mother; the second, with the back of the child inclined toward the sacrum of the mother. The back of the child does not, in either of these cases, look directly forward or backward; but the presentation passes into the pelvis with the breadth of the child in the line of one of the oblique diameters of the brim. When the breech is the presenting part, one of the ischia (usually the most anterior, or that nearest to the pubis) descends lower than its fellow, and first meets the finger of an examiner.

The breech is usually transmitted through the outlet with one hip directed obliquely toward the pubis, and the other toward the sacrum. The shoulders pass the brim with their breadth in the line of the oblique diameter, but in passing the outlet, they have their position changed, being then inclined, the one toward the pubis, and the other toward the sacrum : by this inclination the head is brought through the brim with the forehead towards the sacro-iliac synchondrosis, and the occiput toward the opposite acetabulum. The shoulders having been expelled, the face turns into the hollow of the sacrum, the chin is depressed toward the chest, and so escapes posteriorly ; and, lastly, the vertex passes out from under the pubis.

In the second species, when the face of the child is at first inclined anteriorly, a complete turn is most usually subsequently effected, so as to bring the face into the hollow of the sacrum, as in the first species. Sometimes, however, in these cases, the head, instead of being flexed, is extended, the occiput depressed upon the nape of the neck, and the vertex turns into the hollow of the sacrum. The chin then rests upon the pubis, and the occiput first passes out posteriorly. The above. observations, with the exception of those relating to the passage of the nates, apply accurately to foot and knee presentations.

Presentations of the upper extremities, or side of the body.—In these presentations the child lies transversely across the brim of the pelvis, with its head toward one ilium, and its breech toward the other. A little consideration will show that almost insuperable obstacles oppose its passage while thus situated. In certain cases, however, in which the fœtus is very small, or rendered very pliable by putrefaction, the power of the uterus has been found sufficient to effect its expulsion. This process has been termed by Denman, who particularly noticed it, *spontaneous evolution*, and was first correctly explained by Dr. Douglas of Dublin. It is, in fact, an expulsion of the child with its body doubled together. During its accomplishment, the head rests upon one iliac fossa, the shoulder is driven forwards entirely out of the pelvis, and rises before the pubis, thus making room for the protrusion of the side of the chest into the vulva; again, as this is forced out, the side of the abdomen is pressed after, the body is very much flexed upon itself, until, finally, the breech is, by repeated efforts, expelled over the sacrum. The head, last of all, passes out of the pelvis.

In describing the mechanism employed in head presentations, I have adopted the opinions of Professor Nägele, being convinced of their general correctness. The student, however, is not to be disappointed if he should find himself unable to diagnose the *exact* position of the head in any individual case. It is, in fact, often extremely difficult to do this, and in attempting it, we are by no means warranted in inflicting any pain upon the mother. A failure is of the less consequence, as the whole tenor of the facts ascertained by the excellent observer alluded to, goes to discountenance the idea of its being ever necessary or expedient to change the position of the head.

CHAPTER IV.

ORGANS OF GENERATION—EXTERNAL AND INTERNAL.

A VERY brief description of these parts will be required for the clear understanding of the steps and accidents of labour; it is not, however, necessary to enter into their minute anatomy, with which the reader is presumed to be already sufficiently acquainted. The organs subservient to generation are divided into external and internal.

EXTERNAL ORGANS.—These consist of the mons veneris, the greater labia, the lesser labia or nymphæ, the clitoris, the orifice of the urethra, the hymen, the carunculæ myrtiformes, the fossa navicularis, fourchette, and perineum.

The *mons veneris* is merely the cushion of fat and cellular substance occupying the anterior surface of the os pubis.

The *greater labia* descend upon each side from the mons, become thinner as they pass back toward the anus, at about an inch before which they

unite together.   They are formed of fat and very
distensible cellular substance, and are covered internally with mucous membrane, and externally
with common integument, which, like that covering the mons, is furnished with hairs and sebaceous glands.   The opening between the. labia is
termed the *vulva*, or genital fissure.

The *nymphæ* or *lesser labia* are two folds of
mucous membrane lying within the great labia;
they are united together superiorly immediately
above the clitoris, for which they form a kind of
prepuce.   They become narrower as they pass
along the vagina, about the middle of which they
are lost.   Their use appears to be to increase the
dilatability of the genital fissure, by unfolding
during parturition.

The *clitoris* is placed immediately beneath the
junction of the nymphæ.   It is a small projecting
body, having corpora cavernosa, and erector muscles, resembling those of the penis.   It is endowed
with great sensibility, and is capable of a degree
of erection.

The *orifice of the urethra* is a small pit situated
about three quarters of an inch below the clitoris,
and immediately above the vagina; a small fold
or flap of mucous membrane sometimes projects
from the under margin of the extremity of the
urethra, and gives the orifice somewhat of an up-
ward direction.

While speaking of the orifice of the urethra we may conveniently consider the mode of *introduction of the catheter.* If the operation is to be performed while the woman is in bed, she may lie upon her back, or, what is better, upon her left side, with the hips projecting over the edge of the bed. The left forefinger of the operator is then to be introduced to a short distance (about the length of the first joint) into the vagina, and carried forward to the symphysis pubis. By this measure the urethra will be easily discovered lying between the finger and the pubis. It resembles in feel the corpus spongiosum of the male urethra, but is usually rather thicker. The finger is then to be drawn lightly forward along the urethra, until its tip sinks into the pit marking the orifice, in contact with which it is to be held. The catheter, held loosely between the right thumb and forefinger, is next to be passed along the front of the left forefinger, in a direction somewhat backwards, when it at once slips into the orifice of the urethra. The handle should then be slightly depressed, and the instrument passed on into the bladder; during its introduction the point may catch in one of the mucous lacunæ, upon which it should of course be withdrawn a little, and passed forward with a slight variation of its direction. The urethra is from an inch to two inches long, so that in an ordinary case, where there is no disease, we should expect the urine to flow when the catheter has passed in to the distance of two inches. If it should be necessary, the operation may be performed while the patient sits upon the edge of a chair, the operator kneeling before her, and passing his hand between her thighs. In either case, exposure of the woman's person should be carefully avoided. By adopting the plan just mentioned, instead of that usually directed in books, we shall get rid of the necessity for irritating the clitoris, which, for obvious reasons, is a very considerable improvement.

The *orifice of the vagina* is situated immediately beneath that of the urethra, and in the virgin is usually closed by a fold of the mucous membrane, denominated the *hymen.* This, in the natural state, has a small crescentic opening at the anterior part, through which the menses pass. Occasionally, this opening is wanting, and the membrane is cribriform, or even imperforate.

Carunculæ myrtiformes.—These are three or four wartlike excrescences at the orifice of the vagina, by some supposed to be the remains of the ruptured hymen, but by others said to exist together with it.

The *fossa navicularis* is the name given to the hollow immediately within the posterior commissure of the vulva.

The *fourchette* is the point of union of the labia posteriorly.

The *perineum* is the space between the four-chette and anus. Its extent is from an inch to an inch and a half. It is lined internally by the mucous membrane of the vagina, and externally covered by the skin. Between these there is cellular substance, and some muscular fibres.

INTERNAL ORGANS.—These consist of the vagina,, uterus, Fallopian tubes, and ovaries.

The *vagina* is the membranous canal leading from the vulva to the uterus. It is curved with a concavity forwards, to such an extent that its axis coincides with that portion of the curved line, already mentioned in describing the axis of the pelvis, which describes the axis of the outlet. It is formed of dense cellular membrane, surrounded throughout by numerous nerves and vessels, and at the lower part by muscular fibres, forming a species of sphincter. At about an inch from the orifice (which is its narrowest part), the vessels are collected into a cavernous tissue, denominated the *plexus retiformis*. The internal surface is lined with mucous membrane, which, in the young subject, is arranged into transverse folds or rugæ: it has also many orifices of mucous glands. The superior extremity of the vagina passes up nearly an inch above the os uteri, before its mucous membrane is reflected upon the cervix; this reflection takes place higher behind than before, so that the posterior lip projects more into the canal than the anterior. The anterior wall is connected firmly with the urethra below; and above, by looser cellular substance, with the back of the bladder; this wall in its undisturbed state measures about three inches. The posterior wall (longer) is united to the rectum below; above, it is covered by peritoneum, which forms a cul de sac separating it from the intestine.

The *uterus* is a flattened pyriform body, from two inches and a half to three inches in length, one inch in thickness from before backward, and one inch and a half in breadth at its upper (broad) extremity. It is divided for the purpose of description into the fundus, which is the upper and broadest part; the cervix, or lower extremity; the body, which is that portion between the fundus and cervix; and, lastly, the os uteri or os tincæ, an opening situated at the termination of the cervix, and leading from the vagina to the uterine cavity.

The substance of the uterus is from one third to three quarters of an inch in thickness, and is composed of a peculiar dense, greyish, fibrous tissue, containing abundance of nerves, bloodvessels, and lymphatics. Upon cutting into it, we observe that it contains numerous sinuses. The fibres of the unimpregnated uterus cannot be observed to follow any regular course: they possess all the powers, and most of the appearances, of muscle; although it is a favourite whim with certain anatomists to deny them the name.

Within the solid walls of the uterus a cavity is formed, triangular in that portion contained in the fundus, and with its lower angle prolonged into a narrow canal, which passes through the body and cervix to the os tincæ. At the upper angles on each side are situated the openings of the Fallopian tubes. The whole cavity is lined by mucous membrane continuous with that of the vagina. In the young subject, this is arranged into folds; it has numerous mucous lacunæ, particularly in the cervix.

The os uteri is a transverse slit in the lower extremity of the cervix, varying in length from three to eight lines. It has two lips, which in the virgin are smooth, but, in persons who have had children, they are frequently tuberculated and irregular. In the neighbourhood of the os are situated some follicles, termed the glandulæ Nabothi, which secrete a tough sebaceous matter, and are supposed to be the seat of the cancer that occasionally attacks this part.

The situation of the uterus is near the middle of the pelvis, between the bladder and rectum, its axis coinciding with that of the brim. It is covered on both sides by peritoneum, and is held in situ by the following ligaments. The broad ligaments are merely folds of peritoneum passing off from the sides of the womb to the sides of the pelvic cavity. Each is formed by two layers of peritoneum, between which are situated, at the upper margin, the Fallopian tubes and ovaries, and, lower down, the vessels and nerves of the organ. The anterior and posterior ligaments are also folds of peritoneum passing off respectively upon the bladder and rectum. The round ligaments differ in structure from the others. They pass off on each side from the fundus uteri, close to the insertion of the tubes, and, passing out of the abdomen through the inguinal ring, are lost upon the mons veneris and labia. They are composed of a number of blood-vessels, lymphatics, nerves, and cellular substance, and form a thick round cord. The use of these ligaments has been much disputed. By Sir C. Bell* they have been ingeniously supposed to answer the purpose of tendons, and to furnish a fixed point for the two circular muscles, which he has described as existing at the fundus of the womb. Professor Jörg,† of Leipsic, believes that they communicate sensation from the clitoris to the Fallopian tubes and ovaries at the moment of coition, so as to

* Med. Chir. Trans. vol. iv.
† Handbuch der Geburtshülfe. Leipzig, 1833.

establish a consent of all the parts concerned in generation.

The *Fallopian tubes* are two firm cords, about four inches in length, formed of a spongy cavernous tissue, with blood-vessels, lymphatics, nerves, and probably muscular fibres. They contain a canal, which opens into the fundus of the uterus upon each side, by an opening merely large enough to receive a bristle. The canal enlarges as it runs toward the opposite free extremity, and opens into the cavity of the peritoneum, its termination being surrounded by fimbriæ, and denominated the *morsus diaboli*. The tubes lie in the upper fold of the broad ligaments in a very tortuous manner.

The *ovaries* also lie in the upper fold of the broad ligament behind the tubes. They are flattened whitish bodies, from an inch to an inch and a half long, resembling in appearance and feel the male testes. In the early fœtus this resemblance is so remarkable, that we can sometimes with difficulty distinguish whether the bodies lying in the lower part of the abdomen be actually ovaria or testes. The ovaries are composed of a peculiar cellular tissue, and each contains fifteen or twenty globular cells or vesicles, including a drop of albuminous fluid, and denominated the *vesiculæ Graafianæ*. Each of these vesicles is supposed to contain an ovum, which escapes by the bursting of the peritoneal coat of the ovary at the moment of

conception, leaving behind a small cicatrix. At
the same period an oval glandular body is observed
to be formed in the ovary, about one-third of an
inch in diameter, and resembling much the secre-
tory portion of the kidney. This is named the
corpus luteum. It continues to exist from the
time of conception until three or four months after
parturition; but of its uses we are nearly quite
ignorant.*

In connection with the foregoing description of
the hard and soft parts immediately concerned in
the generative function, it may be interesting to
reflect upon the effects likely to be produced upon
the other organs contained in the pelvis by the
changes resulting from the exercise of this function. The uterus, we have seen, is situated between the bladder and rectum, and accordingly,
as might have been expected, its enlargement
frequently interferes with the action of both these
organs. If the pressure particularly affect the
former viscus, it will be found to occasion frequent micturition and other symptoms of irritation; and when the part pressed upon is the
urethra or neck of the bladder, retention of urine
may be the consequence. In like manner, pressure
upon the rectum will sometimes cause tenesmus,

* Sir E. Home supposed that corpora lutea might exist in
the virgin; but his supposition is not supported by the testimony of other observers.

or constipation, and, by interfering with the free return of the blood, produce or aggravate piles. The great blood-vessels which traverse the pelvis in their course to or from the lower extremities, as well as the numerous lymphatics, are also frequently subjected to interruption of their functions from pressure of the enlarged uterus, to which may be traced the varices and œdema of the limbs so common in pregnancy. The pressure, also, upon the great nerves may satisfactorily explain the numbness and cramps of the legs frequently complained of during labour, and at the latter periods of gestation.

CHAPTER V.

FUNCTIONS OF THE GENERATIVE SYSTEM.

MENSTRUATION.—In every healthy woman, at the age of puberty, a sanguineous discharge occurs from the uterus, and returns regularly every twenty-eight days, excepting at those periods when the woman is either pregnant or giving suck. From the regularity of its return this is denominated the menses or catamenia, and, in ordinary language, ' the monthly courses.' It commences in this country usually about the fourteenth or fifteenth year, and ceases between the forty-fifth and fiftieth. In warm climates, it is said, but I think upon insufficient authority, that it commences and terminates much earlier than in these countries.*

The menstrual discharge, although sanguineous in its appearance, is not pure blood, but strictly a secretion from the uterine vessels. It differs from

* See a paper by Mr. Roberton in the Ed. Med. and Surg. Journal, vol. xxxviii.

blood in being uncoagulable, and containing but a very small quantity of fibrine: although occasionally retained in the uterus for months, in consequence of an imperforate hymen, it has never been observed to coagulate or separate into two portions.

Pure blood may, in consequence of increased action, be poured out along with the menses, and detected by its coagulation; also, coagulable lymph, as in the false membrane of painful menstruation. The secretion may sometimes even be devoid of the usual red colour.

The quantity of the menses varies considerably in different individuals, and, from the slow manner in which it escapes, is not easily estimated; the average quantity, however, in this country appears to be about four ounces. This trickles from the mouth of the uterus (as has been seen in cases of prolapsus of the organ) during a period varying from three to five days.

At the period of the first occurrence of menstruation, a remarkable change takes place in the system of the female. All the organs connected with reproduction then assume a perfect condition. The uterus and vagina enlarge; the external organs become developed and covered with hair, and the breasts increase in size and in perfection of their glandular structure. The whole body also assumes a more characteristically female form; and at the same time the mind ceases to take interest in the pursuits of childhood, and is more or less influenced by the passions of the adult woman.

The use of menstruation is, obviously, closely connected with the function of conception, as it is only during the menstruating period of life that the latter ever takes place. The mode of its action, however, is little explained: most probably it results from the internal surface of the uterus being preserved in a condition capable of secretion, the latter state being necessary to the support and development of an ovum. The causes of its periodical returns, and of the uterine excitement attending its occurrence, appear to me to be not in the remotest degree elucidated by any of the numberless theories that have been offered for its explanation. It would not, therefore, answer any practical end to enter at present into further examination of the subject.

Conception.—This is the chief function of the generative system; and from its nature it is involved in deep obscurity. At present it will be sufficient for our purpose to state simply the facts known, indulging as little as possible in hypotheses, which must be the product rather of fancy than of reason.

In all animals, and even vegetables, in which reproduction is accomplished by the formation of an ovum,* the concurrence of two distinct sets of organs appears to be required. In the lower classes of animals, and in most vegetables, these organs exist together in the same individuals, constituting more or less perfect hermaphrodites. In the higher animals, on the other hand, and in some plants, there is a sexual distinction, the male and female organs being developed in different and distinct individuals. In these it is found that certain rudiments of the new being are prepared in the female, and even brought to a point of considerable perfection (as in birds and those animals which emit their spawn before impregnation), but yet require for their full development the stimulus of the male secretion or semen.

In the human female, the existence of these rudiments in the vesicles of the ovaries, and their passage from thence, through the tubes, to the womb, has been inferred from the following circumstances. In every instance in which an examination has been made shortly after conception, it has been observed that the contents of one or more of these vesicles had been discharged,† and that a cicatrix, marking the point of their exit from the ovary, existed on the peritoneal coat of that body. The formation, at

---

* The seeds of plants are perfectly analogous to ova.

† It is usually found that a drop of blood is effused into the vesicular cavity, which coagulates, and is subsequently absorbed.

the same period, of the corpus luteum in the neighbourhood of the cicatrix (although we are ignorant of its exact uses) also indicates the performance of some special action.   Again, we have, in a morbid state, the occasional development of a fœtus in the ovary, forming a variety of extra-uterine fœtation. That the rudiments pass by the tubes into the uterus may be inferred from the occurrence of another example of extra-uterine fœtation, in which the ovum is arrested in its passage through the tube and partially developed in its canal.   There is also analogical proof to be derived from the experiments of Dr. Haighton,* in which he completely stopped the progress of conception in a rabbit by dividing the tubes within thirty hours from the period of impregnation; but failed in effecting that object when he postponed the division to forty-eight hours from the same period.

As to the manner in which the rudiments escape from the ovary and effect their transit into the womb, we have little information.   By some it is supposed that the vesicle bursts, and that its contents are absorbed by the tube in a fluid state, and so conveyed into the womb.   Mr. Cruikshank's hypothesis was, that it escaped in the form of a perfect cyst; and he conceived that he demonstrated this by opening and pouring distilled vinegar upon the tube of a recently impregnated ani-

* Phil. Trans. vol. lxxxvii.

mal, whereby an egg-like cyst was rendered visible.
This effect, however, might be produced by the
mere coagulation of the albumen probably contained in the fluid rudiments. It is not improbable
that the matter may be absorbed in a fluid form,
and furnished with a cyst composed of the future
amnion and chorion during its transit through the
tube : in support of this conjecture we have an
analogy in the addition of the shell to the ovum
of birds during its passage through the oviduct.

As to the time occupied by these actions, which
may be properly considered as constituting the
process of *conception*, much uncertainty prevails.
It may probably be set down at about a fortnight,
as I believe the ovum has seldom been recognised
in the uterus in less than two or three weeks from
the period of impregnation.

In multiparient animals, and in the human
female who conceives of more than one child, the
number of cicatrices and of corpora lutea in the
ovaries exactly corresponds with the number of
fœtuses in the uterus.

Conception has been hitherto spoken of entirely
with reference to the operations of the female ;
with respect to the part borne by the male, but
little is ascertained with certainty. We are, in fact,
quite ignorant as to the mode in which the semen
effects the awakening of the ovum, which we have
already seen may be brought, in some animals, to

a state of apparent perfection, and expelled from the body, without male aid. It is not even certainly known whether actual contact of the male and female products is an essential requisite of impregnation, or whether this result may not be produced by a mere exhalation or *aura* proceeding from the male semen. In favour of actual contact are some observations of Ruysch, in which he says that he detected semen in the Fallopian tubes of a woman killed in the act of adultery ; the experiments of Dr. Blundell ; * and the analogies of vegetable fecundation, and of the generation of animals whose ova are impregnated after expulsion, in both of which, actual experiments prove the necessity of direct contact. On the other side, we have the unexplained difficulty of effecting contact, and the occasional occurrence of conception while the hymen is perfect, and an insuperable obstacle thus opposed to the entrance of the male organ into the vagina. Upon the whole, the weight of evidence appears to be in favour of actual contact; but where or how effected, we know not. Such is the scanty foundation of facts upon which have been built the innumerable absurd, as well as ingenious though fragile, theories of reproduction.

* Med. Chir. Trans. vol. x.

CHAPTER VI.

GRAVID UTERUS.

COEVAL WITH, and subsequently to conception, many changes take place in the womb and its contents, all of which may be included in the consideration of the gravid uterus. We shall first consider the effects of pregnancy upon the womb itself, and, for the sake of contrast with the un-impregnated state of the organ, we shall examine its size, structure, &c., at the full period of gestation.

At this time it is of an oval shape, somewhat compressed from before backwards, and with the smaller extremity pointed downwards. Its average dimensions are, twelve inches in length, nine in breadth, and six or seven in depth ; these, however, varying according to the size of the fœtus and secundines, and especially to the quantity of the liquor amnii.

The steps by which it attains this size are gradual and regular. Until the end of the third month

it remains within the pelvis. In the fourth it begins to mount above the brim, and then measures
about five inches from the fundus to the beginning
of the neck. At this period the enlargement is
confined to the fundus and body ; but in the fifth
month the cervix begins to be distended, and becomes softer and spongy.

Until the fifth month the weight of the uterus
acts in depressing it into the vagina, so that we
can feel the os tincæ more readily than in the unimpregnated condition : but as the cervix becomes
distended, and the uterus rises into the abdomen,
the vagina is stretched upwards, and the os more
distant from the finger. In the seventh month the
womb reaches usually to the umbilicus, and the
cervix is so much developed that we can often feel
the head of the child through its walls. In the
eighth month the fundus gets to about half way
between the umbilicus and sternum, and the orifice
is on a level with the brim of the pelvis. In the
ninth month the upper extremity of the womb is
very near the ensiform cartilage, the cervix is
completely taken up into the general cavity of
the uterus, and the os changed from a transverse
slit into a round rugous hole, placed without any
projection in the lesser extremity of the organ.

The situation of the full-sized womb is oblique,
with the os directed backwards towards the sacrum, and the fundus forward, so that its axis is

E

nearly identical with that of the brim, being described by an imaginary right line passing from the scrobiculus cordis to the point of the sacrum —a circumstance that requires to be understood, when it is necessary to pass the hand into the uterus.* The gravid womb lies anterior to all the viscera of the abdomen, occupying the whole interval between the iliac bones, and a corresponding space above, as high as the epigastrium.

The structures of the uterus continue essentially the same as in the unimpregnated condition, but undergo a remarkable development. The muscular fibres, which appeared so irregular in the virgin womb, now exhibit a definite arrangement into layers. The outermost of these fibres arise from the round ligaments, and, regularly diverging, spread over the fundus until they unite. According to Sir C. Bell,† the round ligaments are the tendons of these muscles, and serve as fixed points from which they act in bringing the womb down into the pelvis at the commencement of labour, and giving its mouth the proper direction. In the substance of the organ, internal to this layer,

---

* In women who have had many children, this axis is often deviated from, on account of the distensible parietes of the abdomen allowing the uterus to depend forwards. Lateral obliquities also occasionally happen from unequal laxity of the parietes, or from deformities of the spine or pelvis.

† Med. Chir. Trans. vol. iv.

the muscular fibres have a circular direction near the fundus, and a longitudinal near the cervix : they are, however, interwoven together in a very intricate manner ; and when they act fully, must have a very powerful effect in constringing the blood-vessels, which pass between them, and so preventing hemorrhage. Their action, during labour, is to open the os tincæ, and draw it, as it were, over the child's head. The most internal stratum of muscle is arranged with the fibres in two sets of concentric circles, each having the orifice of one of the tubes as its centre. These two muscles, if we may so call them, interweave together at their circumferences, and have proceeding from them, on each side, broad longitudinal bands of fibres, which assist the external muscles in bringing the fundus towards the os, and in drawing the latter over the child's head. The circular portions are supposed to corrugate and diminish the internal surface of the uterus, after the child has been expelled, and so draw it off, as it were, from the placenta, which, having no power of diminishing its own area, must, of course, separate from the surface to which it is attached when the latter is diminished in the way mentioned.

The thickness of the uterine parietes is nearly the same as in the unimpregnated state: in the part to which the placenta is attached, it is perhaps a little thicker.* Its substance throughout is more spongy and vascular, and the sinuses are much more developed than before conception.

The blood-vessels of the womb are much enlarged during gestation, especially in the neighbourhood of the site of the placenta, where the arteries are sometimes as large as the point of the little finger. The veins are proportionally large, and form plexuses, with very free communication. The lymphatics are also very large and numerous.

The nerves, which are derived from the hypogastric and spermatic plexuses of the great sympathetic, and, from the sacral pairs, are said by some (W. Hunter and F. Tiedemann) to be enlarged; a circumstance, however, that has been denied by other observers.†

Contents of the Womb.—These consist of the fœtus, liquor amnii, or waters, and the secundines; all together constituting the ovum. The secundines consist of the funis, placenta, and membranes; the latter being three in number, viz. the decidua, chorion, and amnion.

The *decidua* is the outermost coat of the ovum, and less properly belongs to it than to the uterus, as

---

* The walls of the uterus are sometimes unequally thin in different parts; a knowledge of which circumstance ought to make us particularly cautious when we happen to have our hand in its cavity.

† Jörg, Handbuch der Geburtshülfe.

it is formed in the latter during the process of conception, and before the ovum has descended into its
· cavity. It is also to be found in the womb, in cases
of extra-uterine fœtation, appearing to be, in fact,
a preparation made in the organ for the lodgment
of an expected but absent guest. The exact nature
of this membrane has been much disputed; but it
appears to be, at first, a secretion of organisable
lymph, produced by the vessels of the womb while
under the stimulus of conception.* It is soon
supplied with vessels admitting of being injected
from the uterine arteries, and then assumes the
form of a dense and thick, but friable membrane.
The decidua is not formed in the cervix uteri,
but stretches across its upper part, so as to form
a shut sac in the body and fundus. It also closes
up the openings of the Fallopian tubes on each
side.†

When the ovum passes down, it must, to get
into the womb, remove from the orifice of the
tube the layer which closes it, and in doing so

* In texture and mode of formation it appears to resemble
much the false membrane thrown out in certain inflammations,
as croup, &c.

† Dr. Lee supposes that the decidua is perforated opposite
each tube; but it is scarcely likely that an aperture so minute
as that of the tube would be preserved in a membrane of the
kind. His view also offers a great difficulty in the explanation
of the formation of the decidua reflexa—a subject already
obscure enough. Vide Med. Chir. Trans. vol. xvii.

(*probably*) forms for itself a little bag, having a
neck only equal in diameter to the perforation of
the tube. From the plastic nature of the decidua,
we can easily believe that this bag may increase
in a degree corresponding to the growth of the
ovum, whilst its neck remains of its original size
(that of the tube): it is not detached from any
part of the uterine surface, as some have supposed.
The bag thus formed around the ovum, by the
prolongation and growth of that portion of the
membrane which covered the opening of the tube,
is termed the *decidua reflexa*, in contradistinction
to the portion adherent to the uterus, which is
called the *decidua vera*. The arrangement of
these two portions of the membrane resembles
precisely that of the peritoneum ; the decidua vera
being analogous to the peritoneum lining the
abdominal walls ; and the reflexa, to the same
membrane covering the intestines and other
viscera. It is only at the commencement of
pregnancy that the distinction between the deciduæ vera and reflexa can be perceived, as they
both coalesce when the ovum has attained a certain size. In one situation only are the two
distinct at the time of parturition, and that is
where the placenta intervenes between them :
the membrane (as I have ascertained by repeated
dissections) splits at the edge of the placenta ;
that layer which was the decidua vera passing

over its uterine aspect, while the reflexa is attached to its fœtal surface, interposed between it and the chorion. At this period, the membranes being much condensed, and firmly adherent to the placental surface, it requires some care to demonstrate them.

The use of the decidua appears to be, in the first instance, to afford the means of establishing a connection between the ovum and the uterus: the flocculent vessels of the chorion shooting into it, and (*probably*) anastomosing with the numerous vessels which it has itself derived from the womb. If we may adopt the phraseology of germination, which seems very applicable, we may say that the decidua furnishes the light nutrient soil into which the radicles of the ovum can strike at once, and obtain for it, without difficulty, a supply of nourishing particles sufficient to enable it to elaborate its own system. Later, the decidua assists in the formation of the placenta, in a manner respecting which we shall inquire when speaking of that organ. The membrana decidua, or caduca, has, as its epithets import, but a transitory existence, and is always cast off either along with the ovum, or subsequently to parturition.

The time at which the ovum arrives in the womb is not exactly defined, and has been differently estimated by observers: it has not, I believe, been recognised with certainty before three weeks from the time of impregnation.* When first visible, it is simply a vesicle formed by two concentric membranes, between which and within the inner one is contained a small quantity of clear gelatinous fluid. The outer membrane is the *chorion*. It is, at first, covered with a stratum of flocculent vessels, which strike into the decidua, and are, as it were, the radicles of the ovum. In the later periods of pregnancy, it loses its shaggy appearance, and becomes thin and transparent. It is then adherent to the decidua, covers the placenta (on its inner surface), and is reflected over the cord. Its use appears to be, to contain and strengthen the other parts of the ovum, and to establish a connection with the uterus by means of the decidua.

The *amnion* is a thin, pellucid, but very dense membrane, contained within the chorion, and at first separated from it by the gelatinous fluid already described; but usually towards the close of pregnancy, in close contact with that envelope. It is reflected over the chorion on the placenta and cord.† Its use appears to be as an envelope

* I have known a perfect ovum to be discharged from the uterus exactly seven weeks after *menstruation*. The preparation is in the museum of the medical school at Park-street. It contains an embryo and vesicula umbilicalis with amnion and shaggy chorion, and is altogether not larger than a hazel-nut.

† At the umbilicus both the chorion and amnion pass insensibly into the skin of the fœtus, and are by some supposed

to the embryo, and to secrete the liquor amnii.
Neither of these membranes has been injected in
the human subject; but their vascularity can be
fully ascertained in animals, by injecting from the
fœtal vessels.

The *liquor amnii* is the fluid secreted by and
contained in the amnion. It is composed of
water containing small quantities of albumen,
muriate of soda, and phosphate of lime. It is of
a light straw colour, and has a very peculiar smell.
The liquor amnii varies in quantity, at the full
period of gestation, from half a pint to upwards
of a quart. Its use appears to be, to furnish a
medium in which the fœtus can enjoy a certain
degree of motion, and at the same time be most
effectually protected against external injury. It
has been supposed by some to be a source of nourishment to the fœtus; but, without involving ourselves in the intricacies of this question, it will be
enough to point out the absurdity of any organism
being supposed capable of secreting matter for its
own nourishment. Such would be the case, however, if the liquor amnii served this purpose, as it
can only be produced from the fœtal vessels; the
amnion having no vascular connection with the
mother. We shall now take a brief notice of the
fœtus, the main object for which all this apparatus

to be, in original formation, identical with the cutis and epi-
dermis.

is constructed; and lastly, examine its means of
support while in the uterus, and the organs acces-
sory thereto.

The Fœtus.—After the lapse of a period, not as
yet certainly ascertained, the simple vesicle of
early pregnancy is found, upon close inspection,
to contain a minute opaque body attached to its
inner surface by a slender and very short filament.
When first seen, this corpuscle appears curved
into a semicircle, and without any distinction of
parts. In a short time a distinction is evident
between the head and body; but the fundamental
part appears always to be the spine. In the second month, the extremities begin to bud out, as
it were, from the body; and between the lower
limbs the spine projects somewhat in the form of
a tail. At the same time the face, and organs of the
cavities sprout out from the concave side of the
corpuscle. The eyes also appear, and subsequently
the mouth, nostrils, and openings of the ears. In
the course of the second and third months, the
genitals are formed, but present very little difference in the different sexes, the penis and clitoris
being nearly of equal size, and the testes, which
remain in the abdomen until the seventh or eighth
month, much resembling the ovaria. Ossification
commences about the seventh or eighth week.
During the third and fourth month the nose, lips,
eyelids, and ears are forming, and the parietes of

the abdomen are completed, so as to include the intestines, which previously formed a sort of hernia in the commencement of the funis. The extremities continue to grow in a branch-like manner, and to form at their termination the fingers and toes. About the end of the fifth month, the fœtus has nearly assumed its perfect form, and has then chiefly to increase in size. It still, however, differs considerably from the child: the testicles are in the abdomen, the eyelids coherent, and the pupil closed by a membrane called *membrana pupillaris*.

Even at the full period, the fœtus differs remarkably from the child in many of its organs, and especially in those concerned in circulation. Into these differences (which are dwelt upon in every system of physiology) it will not be necessary, at present, to enter farther than merely to call to mind the peculiarities of the circulating system. It is to be recollected, that, from the want of atmospheric air, the lungs are incapable of performing their function; and, accordingly, a vicarious organ is supplied in the placenta. From this the renovated blood is sent through the umbilical vein to the inferior cava, supplying, as it passes, large branches to the liver. The portion of the umbilical vein which passes through the fissure of the liver is denominated the *ductus venosus*, and exists merely as a cord in the breathing child. From the inferior cava the blood passes in the regular course into the right auricle, and from thence part of it goes through the foramen ovale (which closes after birth) directly into the left auricle; from thence into the left ventricle, and so by the aorta into the general circulation. Another portion of the blood in the right auricle passes in the ordinary course into the right ventricle, and thence into the pulmonary artery; but as the uninflated lungs are not capable of receiving it, a passage, termed the *ductus arteriosus* (not pervious after birth), conveys it into the aorta, where it joins the blood which has passed through the foramen ovale, and is distributed along with it throughout the body. From the iliac arteries, however, two branches, denominated the hypogastric, pass off upon the back of the bladder, ascend to the umbilicus, and then become the arteries of the cord: these convey a considerable portion of blood from the descending aorta back to the placenta, for the purpose of renovation. The hypogastric arteries degenerate into cords in the breathing child.

The body of the fœtus is covered with a whitish sebaceous matter, called the *vernix caseosa*: the use of this is, probably, to protect the skin against the effects of long immersion in the liquor amnii. The average weight of the fœtus at the full period is about seven pounds: it is sometimes, however, as much as twelve pounds: the average joint weight of twins is eleven pounds. In the gravid uterus

the fœtus is packed into the smallest possible
space, its chin depressed upon the breast, its
legs flexed upon the thighs, and the latter upon
the abdomen, the arms crossed upon the chest,
or placed with the hands upon the sides of the
face.

The *funis* is composed of three vessels, the two
arteries just mentioned which bring the impure
blood to the placenta, and the umbilical vein
which carries it back from that organ to the body:
the vein is considerably larger than the arteries.
None of these vessels send off any branches until
they are entering the placenta, when the arteries
anastomose by a cross branch. They do not,
however, run a straight course, but are twisted
spirally together, and also are tortuous, forming
coils upon themselves. The substance of the cord
consists of a cellular web, filled with a gelatinous
matter, and covered firmly by the chorion and
amnion. In this gelatinous tissue the vessels are
imbedded, and thus very effectually preserved from
injury. Owing to this provision, knots are frequently formed upon the cord, without in the
least interrupting the circulation. Besides the
arteries and vein, the cord contains a rudiment of
the urachus and the omphalo-mesenteric vessels
and vitelline pedicle, structures which shall be subsequently alluded to. The existence of nerves
and lymphatics in the funis has been denied by

most anatomists; but Sir Everard Home has alleged that he discovered the former by means of
the microscope; and Dr. V. Fohmann,* of Lüt-
tich, asserts that he has been able to inject ab-
sorbent vessels with mercury, and that they are
very numerous both in the cord and placenta.
The testimony of these gentlemen has not yet, I
believe, been corroborated; † and I fear that at
least Dr. F.'s argument (like many an excellent
one) is injured by too much proof, as he is not
satisfied with stating the existence of those vessels, but proceeds to show that, except the vein
and arteries, the funis contains *nothing* else but
absorbents.   The length of the cord varies,
but is usually about two feet: it is frequently,
when too long, twisted round the neck of the
child.

The *placenta* is the most important of all the
uterine organs of the fœtus, without which neither
growth nor subsistence can continue.   It has
various forms in different animals, but, in the
human subject, is a flat circular body, about six
inches in diameter, and about one inch and a half
in thickness at the centre, becoming thinner toward the circumference.   Usually in the centre,

---

* Zeitschrift für Physiologie, 4ter Bd. 1832.

† Since the above was written, Dr. Montgomery, of Dublin,
has succeeded in repeating Dr. Fohmann's injection in the
funis.

but sometimes at or near the edge, we find the insertion of the funis, whose vessels immediately ramify in a divergent manner upon the surface of the organ. The placenta gives to the touch a peculiar rough fleshy feel, which the student will do well to make himself familiar with, that he may be enabled to recognise it while in the uterus. The external, or uterine, surface is covered with a thin layer of decidua, intimately connected with its substance. Under the decidua the placenta is divided into lobes, the surfaces of which have somewhat of a rough, spongy appearance; and by some it is said that there are defined openings to be observed, leading through the decidua into the substance.* Much dispute has arisen as to the connection of this surface with the uterus. Hunter supposed that large vessels passed directly from the mother into cells in the placenta. A different opinion was entertained by the Monros,† and has been lately very ably advocated by Dr. Robert Lee. These gentlemen deny that any connection exists between the uterus and placenta, except, perhaps, by small nutrient vessels. Later still, Dr. H. Ley‡ has had an opportunity of accurately examining a gravid uterus, and he corroborates the

* Dr. H. Ley in Med. Gaz. vol. xii.

† Med. Essays, vol. ii.; and Essays and Observ. Phys. and Lit. vol. i.

‡ Med. Gaz. vol. xii.

account of Hunter, which is also supported by the testimony of Professor Burns. As yet, I think, we must consider the question as unsettled, although probabilities certainly appear to be against the notion that any very large vessels pass directly between the two parts. The internal, or fœtal, surface of the placenta is not, like the other, divided into lobes, nor has it the same spongy, glandular appearance, but is formed of an immense congeries of vessels, together with cellular substance and a number of white filaments, the nature of which does not appear to be understood: it is covered by a thin layer of decidua, which is very intimately connected to it, and by the chorion and amnion.

The internal structure of the placenta has been the subject of much dispute. It can be injected freely from the vessels of the cord; and it was supposed by William Hunter that injections could also be thrown from the uterine vessels into cells in its substance. From these circumstances, and from the fact of distinct uterine and fœtal portions actually existing in the placenta of many animals, Hunter inferred, that in the human female it is also composed of two parts: the one cellular, communicating with the uterus by a direct passage of vessels; the other vascular, and being, in fact, the ramifications of the umbilical vessels. From the result of his injections, he inferred further, that these portions had no vascular intercommunication. By others it has been stated, that no passage of injection can be effected from the uterine vessels into the placenta, except as the result of extravasation, and that there are no cells whatsoever in its structure, but that it is entirely composed of the fœtal vessels. From the best consideration that I have been able to give the subject, this latter view certainly appears to me to be the most correct; but I am far from thinking that the question has been ultimately set at rest. It is probable that the purposes of the *glandulæ uterinæ*, or maternal placenta of animals, are effected in the human womb by a peculiar development of that portion of the uterine wall to which the placenta is attached, and not by any contrivance in the substance of the latter organ. The testimony with respect to the existence of nerves and lymphatics in the placenta is the same as was mentioned in favour of the presence of the same organs in the funis; that of Sir E. Home and Fohmann. Dr. Fohmann asserts that the lymphatics convey nourishing material from the mother through the cord to the iliac glands, and thence into the system of the fœtus.

The uses of the placenta appear to be in some degree analogous to those of the lungs and stomach of the breathing animal. The blood passes into it from the hypogastric arteries, and,

F

after a very free circulation through it, returns by the umbilical vein directly to the heart. This circulation continues until respiration is established, when it ceases spontaneously, and any interruption of it, before the latter process has commenced, is immediately fatal. From these facts, we are warranted in inferring that a change necessary to life (probably oxygenisation) is effected in the placenta, although the nature of that change is obscure, and the relative properties of the blood in the umbilical arteries and veins are not at all known. That the organ in question not only re-vivifies the blood, but also elaborates new vital fluid, thus performing a function analogous to that of the stomach, can only be inferred from the absence of any other source from whence the fœtus could obtain materials for growth and support.

With respect to the manner in which the placenta is formed, all is obscurity ; but the following appears to me to be a probable conjecture. In speaking of the decidua reflexa, I have mentioned the probability of its being formed by the ovum, in its entrance into the womb, pushing before it that portion of decidua vera which covered the opening of the tube, and so forming a bag, the neck of which would remain attached to the tube, while it would itself (from its plastic nature) increase in a ratio with the increase of the ovum. In a short time this bag of decidua reflexa would be pressed against some part of the uterine wall (most probably in the vicinity of the fundus), and there meeting with a membrane exactly similar to itself (the decidua vera), a vascular union would very soon be established. The result of this union would soon be a minute anastomosis of vessels, and a formation of membranous tissue to support them, between the two deciduæ, and, in process of time, the elaboration of a perfect placenta.

We have now disposed of the principal contents of the gravid uterus, and shall merely allude to two structures, to which great importance has been attached by some, but the uses of which, in reality, are very imperfectly understood.

The *vesicula umbilicalis* is a small body, not exceeding in size a small pea, which lies between the chorion and amnion, near the margin of the placenta. It is connected with the intestines of the fœtus, by a duct denominated the vitelline pedicle, which runs along the funis; and is also connected with the mesenteric vessels by an artery and vein, called the omphalo-mesenteric, which accompany the vessels of the cord through the umbilicus. The vesicle contains a small quantity of a kind of oily matter, supposed to perform a part in the early nutrition of the embryo : but the fact is, we know nothing about the matter.

Allantois. — By some persons a lutcierated membrane is described as existing between the chorion and amnion, which they describe as analogous to the allantoid of brutes, and from which they say the urachus proceeds along the cord to the fundus of the bladder. By others, the existence of an allantoid in the human subject is altogether denied, and the urachus is considered merely as a rudimental type of the same organ in animals. The use of the allantoid has been generally supposed to be for a reservoir for the urine of those animals in which it exists. Velpeau, who admits the existence of some structure of the kind in the human subject, supposes that it serves some unknown purpose in the early nutrition of the fœtus.

CHAPTER VII.

A VERY important duty frequently devolves upon the practitioner of midwifery, when he is called upon to determine as to the actual existence of pregnancy in any individual case. It is necessary for him to be able to solve this question in the ordinary routine of his business, in order that he may be able to inform his patients of their exact condition. Again, it is frequently put to him, when there is a doubt as to whether certain symptoms are traceable to disease, or to a gravid state of the womb; and, thirdly, his judgment upon this point may be required in the management of some of the gravest concerns of public justice. The question, however, is often much easier asked than answered; and it therefore becomes us to examine carefully those signs that indicate the pregnant condition. The chief of these are:—1. amenorrhœa, or suppression of the menses; 2. sympathies of other parts with the irritation of the uterus, viz.

of the stomach, producing nausea and vomiting ; of the nervous system, giving rise to irritability of temper, anomalous pains, salivation, &c. ; and of the breasts, causing a painful development of their glandular substance, and a change of colour in the areola surrounding the nipple ; 3. the motion of the fœtus in utero (denominated quickening); 4. alterations in the uterus as to its general size, and as to the condition of particular parts, as the os and cervix ; and 5. the auscultatory evidence as to the pulsations of the fœtal heart, and the placentary sound.

Suppression of the Menses.—This sign is one which we must take entirely upon trust from the report of the patient. It may also be a morbid symptom ; so that its existence *per se* is no evidence of pregnancy. On the other hand, the presence of the menses affords merely presumptive proof of the non-existence of the same state, as it is well known that discharges similar to the menstrual may occur regularly during gestation. We should only value it, therefore, in connection with other symptoms ; but if such exist, and amenorrhœa continues without loss of health, we have, at all events, good grounds for suspicion.

Sympathies of the Stomach.—Nausea and vomiting are very constant attendants upon conception, occurring sometimes immediately after impregnation, but generally about the third or

fourth week, and usually ceasing at the time of
quickening. As these symptoms may be occasioned by many other causes, they are obviously
not conclusive signs of pregnancy : when they arise
from this state, they usually occur at the time of
the day when the woman, in leaving her bed,
changes from the horizontal to the erect posture,
and are therefore called ' morning sickness.' In
ordinary cases the vomiting is attended with little
general disturbance, hunger being felt immediately
after the stomach has been emptied ; but, in some
instances, the irritability continues throughout the
whole day during the entire period of gestation,
and is attended with much distress.

Sympathies of the Nervous System.—These are
of little importance, conveying, of themselves, no
practical information. I have known salivation,
which I can consider merely as a nervous sympathy, to continue profusely during the greater
part of a pregnancy, and to cease immediately after
parturition, without being productive of any bad
effects. Under this head we may, perhaps, also
include the capriciousness of appetite and temper
often observed in pregnant women, and the anomalous pains, toothaches, &c., of which they
occasionally complain. Neither am I aware of any
other *set of words* which we can use by way of
explanation of the changes that occur in the circulating and urinary systems. The urine has been

observed to contain a peculiar milky deposit, and
the pulse, during gestation, is commonly very
rapid; I have known it beat 140 in a minute, in
a healthy woman.   The popular notion, that the
blood is always buffed during pregnancy, is, according to my opinion (founded upon numerous
observations), merely a popular fallacy.

Sympathies of the Breasts.—Very often the
earliest symptom of pregnancy is a sensation of
weight, pain, and swelling of the breasts.   It frequently occurs in the first month, and before the
time when the non-appearance of the menses
would give reason to suspect the state of the case.
Shortly after conception (about the second or
third month), some remarkable changes take place
in these organs.   They grow larger and firmer,
and their glandular structure becomes evidently
more developed, sometimes so much so as to be
attended with a secretion of milk.   At the same
time, the areola around the nipple becomes usually
darker in colour, moister upon its surface, and
covered with a number of small papillæ.   The
latter changes are considered by many, and, I
believe, with reason, as very certain signs of pregnancy : they apply, however, with more force to
first cases, as the areola, after having been once
changed, seldom resumes its virgin characters so
perfectly as to enable us to recognise, with facility,
subsequent alterations.   We have also to recollect

that, during lactation, the areola retains the same
appearances, and that, in some instances of actual
pregnancy, these may *not* be observable at all.
With respect to the increase in the size of the
breasts, we must be careful to distinguish knotty
glandular development, which is the true sign of
pregnancy, from fatty enlargement, which not
unfrequently perplexes our diagnosis, especially
when we have to deal with a patient who has
been married at a late period of life. Such individuals are apt to become suddenly corpulent,
in consequence of the change effected by marriage
both in their moral and physical constitution;
and, being usually very anxious for heirs, they
often mistake the fatty increase of their breasts
for a certain indication of pregnancy.

Quickening.—By this is understood the first
sensation, on the part of the mother, of the motions
of the child in utero. It occurs usually about the
sixteenth week,* sometimes a little earlier or later,
and is by some supposed to happen always at the
time when the uterus first rises out of the pelvis
into the abdomen. I believe this ascent sometimes
occurs rather suddenly, and is under such circumstances attended with a feeling of nausea and

---

* Some women come to very accurate conclusions respecting
the period of their labour from observing the time of quickening.
I have heard women assert that they quickened at different, but
regular periods, with boys and girls.

faintness; but I rather think it has no necessary connection with the woman's sensation of the first motions of the child, as I have repeatedly felt the uterus in the abdomen long before any quickening had taken place. Great value must be attached to this sign of pregnancy, when women have no motive for misrepresentation, and have had experience of former pregnancies; but, even under such circumstances, we find that they are themselves occasionally deceived, mistaking the motions of air in their own intestines, or spasms of their abdominal muscles, for actions of the fœtus. In many instances the pressure of the cold hand of the accoucheur, during examination, will excite the child to motion; and we might then suppose that no loop was left to hang a doubt upon; but, as if to remind us that we are very fallible, we find cases related (for instance, that of the celebrated Joanna Southcote), in which medical men erroneously supposed that they had felt these movements. In estimating the negative value of absence of quickening, we have to recollect that a dead child may be in the womb, and, of course, motionless; and that some anomalous cases are related, in which quickening never became perceptible, either to the mother herself, or to other examiners.

Enlargement of the Abdomen.—This is the sign which, in doubtful cases, oftenest attracts the attention of casual observers. During the first three months, the abdomen is not at all enlarged (unless accidentally from the presence of air in the intestines); but is, on the contrary, rather flattened, and the umbilicus appears as if dragged inwards. About the end of the third month, however, the abdomen begins to increase in size, and continues gradually enlarging until towards the end of the ninth month; when it sinks and lessens, preparatory to the occurrence of labour. The umbilicus, near the end of gestation, is raised to a level with the surrounding skin, and sometimes even projects.

An enlargement of the abdomen, leading to a supposition of pregnancy, may be occasioned by ascites, tympanitis, fat, or morbid tumors. The diagnostic marks are, under the two first diseases, the presence of their peculiar symptoms, and the absence of the firm, regular outline of the gravid uterus. When the increase is fatty, we have, in place of the condition last mentioned, a soft and yielding state of the abdomen, which admits of our pressing the closed hand backwards, towards the spine. Morbid tumors must be diagnosed by their history and peculiar symptoms: they frequently, however, give rise to much difficulty; and, as well as the other mentioned causes of enlargement, often require an investigation into all the marks, to enable us to distinguish the true nature of the case.

When investigating the cause of an enlarged abdomen, we are obliged to resort to manual examination externally, and perhaps internally (*per vaginam*). To facilitate the external examination we must relax the abdominal walls as much as possible, by placing the woman on her back, with the shoulders raised, and knees drawn up, and engage her in conversation, so as to prevent her from keeping the muscles in a tense condition. When the patient is fat, the diagnosis is much obscured; but if this be not the case, we shall probably be able to recognise the firm, rounded outline of the womb, of a size corresponding with the supposed period of pregnancy. Percussion may be used with advantage in these cases. If a tympanitic sound be elicited by this method of investigation, it will then be highly probable that the swelling is not attributable to any solid tumor, such as a gravid uterus, but to the existence of flatus in the intestines. An internal examination may be made while the patient is lying upon her left side, with her hips projecting over the edge of a bed or couch, and her back towards the examiner; or while she is in an upright posture. One or two fingers (previously oiled) are to be passed gently into the vagina, and carried upwards, so as to investigate the following points.

State of the Os and Cervix Uteri.—It has been already shown that, about the fifth or sixth months, considerable changes take place in the cervix ; and accordingly it is about this period that we derive the most certain information from an internal examination. This part of the womb, not being distended by the ovum during the first months, is pressed downwards by the increased weight of the fundus, and then projects rather more than usual into the vagina; but, at the termination of the fifth month, it begins to be taken up into the general cavity, and, therefore, becomes shorter and less prominent. The cervix continues to be shortened, until, at the ninth month, its canal is completely merged in the general cavity of the uterus; and we then have no projection whatever, but merely feel the os uteri as a rugous circular opening in the lower extremity of the womb, the wall of which is spread evenly over the head of the child. From the first periods of gestation, the os uteri itself undergoes certain changes: it appears to become the seat of a more active circulation, losing its former gristly elastic feel, and becoming softer, and more spongy. During the first five months it is easily felt; but, according as the cervix shortens, and the fundus leans more forward against the anterior wall of the abdomen, it is inclined more backwards and upwards towards the promontory of the sacrum, and at the termination of the ninth month is often out of reach of the finger. That the tumor felt in the abdomen is identical

with that felt per vaginam, we may satisfy ourselves by placing one hand on the abdomen, and
ascertaining that motion is communicable from it
to the fingers of the other hand pressing against
the os and cervix.   This sensation, however, might
be occasioned by a uterus morbidly enlarged, or
one which contained other substances besides an
ovum, as, for example, hydatids; and to obviate
such a deception, the mode of examination called
by the French *ballottement* has been devised.   To
perform this we must introduce one or two fingers
per vaginam, the woman being in an upright
posture; and while the other hand upon the abdomen presses down the womb, we tap quickly against
the cervix, so as to jerk up the fœtus, which floats
for a second or two in the liquor amnii, and
then falls lightly on the finger.   If this circumstance occurs, it is, of course, proof positive
of the existence of a fœtus; but it is not
always that we can succeed in the trial.   Besides
the changes in the size and texture of the os and
cervix uteri, a remarkable alteration in the colour
of the mucous membrane covering these parts and
lining the vagina takes place.   From the usual
bright red hue it changes to a deep dark red, almost
assuming a purple tinge.   This begins early, about
the fourth month, increases in intensity until delivery, and remains for two or three weeks after
that has taken place.

Auscultatory evidence.—The application of auscultation to the investigation of pregnancy constitutes a very valuable addition to our means of
diagnosis. Two sounds may generally be recognised in the uterus during the latter periods of
gestation. The placental soufflet, or *bruit placen-
taire*, is heard for the first time when the uterus,
having risen out of the pelvis, has come into contact with the abdominal walls, *i. e.* about the
fourth month. It consists of a low murmuring
or cooing sound, generally likened to that produced by blowing over the mouth of a phial, and
is synchronous with the pulse of the mother. Its
situation is in that part of the womb to which the
placenta is attached, and varies, of course, in different individuals. A sound perfectly similar has
been found to exist in some morbid tumors of
the abdomen.* The second sound is that of the
fœtal heart. This can seldom be heard until after
the fifth month, and even then not generally with
much distinctness. It consists of regular double
pulsations, varying in rapidity, but always considerably quicker than the pulse of the mother.
The sound resembles the ticking of a watch
heard through a couple of thick pillows when the
head is laid on them. The most likely place to

---

* Mr. Cusack lately directed my attention to a *soufflet*,
perfectly similar to the placental, which issued from an enlarged
thyroid gland.

find it is in one of the iliac regions; but its situation, of course, changes with the position of the child, and in consequence of these changes it may be heard, then lost, and subsequently heard again. This sound, when once recognised, can scarcely be mistaken, and it affords indubitable evidence of pregnancy. Its absence, however, does not prove the contrary, as it may exist, and elude our observation; or there may be a dead fœtus, when it will, of course, be wanting.

From all that has been said respecting the individual signs of pregnancy, it must be obvious that none of them, singly, affords means for a certain diagnosis. The most important information is certainly to be derived from internal examination, and from the employment of auscultation; but even these do not always furnish conclusive evidence, and it is only from a careful enquiry into all the marks, and a collation of them with each other, that we can usually be warranted in giving a decisive opinion, either negatively or affirmatively. In many cases, also, the difficulties in the way of the practitioner will be much enhanced by the existence, at the same time, of pregnancy and disease (for example, ascites or morbid tumors): he will then, perhaps, have at once to deal with both positive and negative signs, and should never give an opinion without the most patient, and, if necessary, protracted, consideration.

Duration of pregnancy.—It is very difficult to come to *perfectly* exact conclusions as to the duration of pregnancy, but the most generally received notion, and which I believe to be very correct, assigns nine calendar months, or between 39 and 40 weeks, as the term. It is not improbable that, occasionally, labour may occur a day or two earlier or later; but there is no perfect certainty upon the subject.

Reckoning, or the computation of the duration of pregnancy, is kept in three ways. First, from the period of conception, which if known leads to the most accurate results; but, of course, it can only be ascertained under very peculiar circumstances. Secondly, from a cessation of the menses, which is subject to a trifling inaccuracy, as the woman may have conceived immediately after the last menstruation, or immediately before the next period. For this debateable time, they usually allow two weeks, and so reckon upon being delivered 42 weeks from their last menstruation. Thirdly, women frequently check the last mode of reckoning by the period of their quickening, which they generally calculate to occur 24 weeks before labour.

CHAPTER VIII.

NATURAL LABOUR.

FROM the sketch which has been given of the anatomy and physiology of the gravid uterus, it must be obvious that the separation from that organ of the foreign substances (so to speak) contained within it, will involve a difficult and elaborate process. Mere expulsion of these substances, however, is not all that is required; provision must be further made for a perfect restoration of the parts concerned in gestation to their ordinary unimpregnated condition. These two purposes are effected chiefly by a series of involuntary contractile efforts taking place in the muscular fibres of the uterus, assisted by voluntary action of the abdominal muscles and diaphragm, and by a *disposition* to dilate, which simultaneously occurs, in the birth passages. In natural parturition, the uterus, by contractions frequently repeated, separates the attachment between its own walls and the ovum, and completely expels the latter; at the same time, its fibres constringe the large vessels which pass between them, so effectually, as often to prevent the escape of even a drop of blood. Finally, by a quiet continuance of the contracting process, the organ is in no very long time reduced to its natural size and condition. The contractions of the uterine fibres are invariably attended with suffering to the woman, and have thence been called '*pains*;' the whole process, from its difficulty, and the muscular exertions required in it, has been appropriately termed '*labour*.'

The determining cause of natural labour cannot be explained: it appears as if the ovum possessed a power of existence within the uterus for a definite period, at the expiration of which it becomes to the latter as a foreign body. This, however, is merely a form of speech, as we are ignorant of the changes which cause it constantly to become a stimulant to the uterine walls at the termination of nine months: all we know is, that at this precise period gestation is completed and labour begins.

Every author upon midwifery adopts a division of the subject of labour, and definitions suitable to his own views; but as I am not aware that one of these is much more practical than another, I shall content myself with those of Dr. Denman, which possess the merit of simplicity, and of being at the same time sufficiently comprehensive: we shall, then, consider all the phenomena of parturition, regular and irregular, under the heads of *natural, difficult, preternatural,* and *anomalous* labours.

Natural labour Dr. Denman defines to be, ' one in which the head of the child presents, which is completed in twenty-four hours, and requires no artificial assistance.' Professor Burns adds the condition of labour not occurring until the full period of gestation. Mauriceau requires that the child should be alive ; and Drs. Cooper and Power restrict the time for a natural labour, the former to twelve, and the latter to six, hours.*

Premonitory signs of labour.—Some days before the commencement of labour, a remarkable subsidence of the abdomen and diminution in the size of the woman ordinarily takes place. This is occasioned partly by the sinking of the cervix uteri (with its contents) into the brim of the pelvis, and partly, perhaps, by the gradual closure of the uterine walls, previous to their taking on active contractile efforts. It is a favourable occurrence,

---

* In 839 cases of labour, which occurred in the Wellesley Institution, 347 terminated in - 6 hours.

300	ditto	-	12 hours.
87	ditto	-	18 hours.
59	ditto	-	24 hours.
37	ditto	-	48 hours.
3	ditto	-	56 hours.
5	ditto		60 hours.
1	ditto	-	72 hours.

as it indicates room in the pelvis, and a disposition to act upon the part of the uterus. About the same time, the woman becomes restless and anxious: if her bladder or rectum be irritable, she perhaps suffers from strangury or tenesmus in a greater or lesser degree; an increased mucous discharge takes place from the vagina, and she may have flying pains and stitches through the loins and abdomen. This is a common course, but in some instances labour begins at once, without any warning whatsoever.

It is not unusual for the flying pains which have been just mentioned to occur many days before labour and to assume a degree of severity which induces the attendants to suppose that that process has actually commenced; they are then called 'false pains,' and require some attention on the part of the practitioner, to enable him to distinguish them from the 'true pains.' They often arise from over-fatigue of the abdominal muscles, or from accumulations of air or fæces in the intestines, and, as they occur irregularly, without producing any effect upon the os uteri, and weary the patient unprofitably, they sometimes require medical treatment. A mild aperient of rhubarb or castor oil, where the bowels are confined, followed by an anodyne draught,* or the latter

---

* Tinct. Opii., gts. xxv. vel xxx.

by itself, when the former is not needed, will very generally afford relief. The best mode of enabling a student to mark the distinction between the true and false pains, will probably be to impress upon him just notions of the character of the former, which we shall now proceed to consider.

The suffering from true pains is usually referred to the back and loins, whence it shoots round to the upper part of the thighs; or at first, perhaps, it commences in the lower region of the abdomen, and darts backward to the loins through the cervix of the uterus. True pains recur with perfect regularity, the interval between any two of them being equal, or gradually and regularly diminishing as labour advances.* If we place our finger upon the os uteri during a true pain, we find that it is tightened and contracted in some degree, more or less, according to the strength of the uterine action; when that ceases it relaxes, and will be found more dilated than it was before the pain commenced. When the dilatation has somewhat advanced, the membranes can be distinguished pressing into the opening during a pain.

A marked difference exists in the character of the pains, according to the period of the labour:

* The interval between pains may vary in different cases from one minute to thirty or forty, according to the activity of the uterus.

at first their operation is chiefly to dilate the os uteri, and for this purpose the uterine fibres are themselves sufficient; accordingly there is no voluntary muscular action. From the peculiar suffering which these pains occasion, they are termed 'grinding' or 'cutting' pains, and during their occurrence the woman usually expresses her sensations by shrill, acute cries. When the os tincæ has been dilated to a certain extent, the pains (which are then termed 'bearing') are accompanied by a strong expulsive effort, and to render this more effective, the woman instinctively brings her abdominal muscles into powerful action. In accomplishing this, she must hold in her breath, and of course can utter no complaint, until the termination of the pain, when she gives vent to her sufferings by a deep, protracted groan. An experienced ear will often receive accurate information as to the state of the labour from the character of the cries; but, in many cases, no expression of suffering will escape the patient until the moment at which the head is passing the external parts, when a scream of agony is usually uttered, which no one who has once heard it will be likely to mistake.

When pains exist which differ remarkably from the foregoing description, especially in having an irregular interval, and producing no dilating effect upon the os uteri, we may safely consider them as 'false,' and as giving no evidence of the existence of labour.

The course of a natural labour has been divided into stages—differently by different authors. The division we shall adopt is that of Dr. Denman, into three stages, merely because it is the most familiar, and is not less practical than any other I have met with. The first stage includes 'all the circumstances which occur, and all the changes made, from the commencement of the labour to the complete dilatation of the os uteri, the rupture of the membranes, and the discharge of the waters;' the second, 'those which occur between that time and the expulsion of the child;' and the third, 'all the circumstances which relate to the separation and expulsion of the placenta.'

The premonitory signs already mentioned having probably shown themselves, the first stage commences by the occurrence of sharp pains in the loins or abdomen. These recur, as has been stated, at regular intervals; and, after they have lasted for some time, the increased mucous discharge from the vagina will be observed to contain some slimy matter tinged with blood. This is denominated by nurses 'a show,' or perhaps 'a red appearance:' it consists of the blood discharged by a rupture of the small vessels connecting the sides of the cervix uteri to the membrana decidua which crosses it; and of the plug or operculum of inspissated mucus which closes the womb during gestation : in some instances, the latter will be discharged in its perfect plug-like form. The pains at first are 'grinding,' and have a long interval; but the latter gradually shortens, while the pains themselves become longer. If we examine *per vaginam*, the os tincæ will be found to contract slightly during each pain, and, relaxing afterwards, by degrees to become more and more permanently dilated. As this occurs, the bag of membranes is protruded into the opening, and, acting as a soft wedge, materially assists in the dilating process. Each pain forces more of the sac into the vagina, until at last it presses upon the external parts ; when, the dilatation of the os tincæ being complete, the membranes burst, and the liquor amnii is discharged; so terminating the first stage.

During this stage a slight degree of febrile excitement generally exists; the patient is anxious and desponding, with a raised pulse and flushed face: sometimes there is considerable fever, with shiverings, headache, thirst, &c. In almost every instance there is nausea and vomiting, arising from the close sympathy which exists between the stomach and os uteri. This is usually most strongly marked about the time when the full dilatation of the os uteri takes place. Some women sleep between every pain throughout the whole course of their labour.

In cases of first children, the dilating stage commonly occupies several hours (from six to thirty-six); but in some persons, especially those who have had a number of children, the os uteri opens with very few pains and little difficulty. Occasionally the waters are discharged too early, —an occurrence generally followed by uterine action so violent as to exhaust the patient before the mouth of the womb is opened sufficiently to admit of the passage of the fœtus, thereby rendering the subsequent progress of the labour tedious and unfavourable.*

Second stage.—After the waters have been discharged, the true bearing or expulsive pains more decidedly set in; the interval becomes shorter, while the uterine action continues a longer period, and is accompanied with more voluntary exertion.

The head of the child is now driven through the os uteri into the vagina, passing the brim with the saggittal suture corresponding to one of the

---

* This consequence would appear to follow only when uterine action comes on immediately (say in twenty-four or forty-eight hours) after early rupture of the membranes. I have known the accident to occur days and even weeks before labour, and yet the latter to be easy and natural.

oblique diameters. As the pains continue, the face is turned into the hollow of the sacrum, and the head presses upon the perineum, the uterine efforts appearing to act upon the child as if they would force it backwards through the latter part.* At this time, if there be any fæces in the rectum, they are expelled during the pain; or if the intestine be empty, the woman mistakes the pressure upon it for an inclination to go to stool. By degrees, however, the head is guided along the inclined planes of the sacrum and ischia, until the vertex is forced under the arch of the pubis, and appears externally between the labia. From this position it recedes upon the cessation of the pain, and is again protruded by the next effort, the retraction and protrusion being repeated a greater or lesser number of times, according to the more or less dilatable condition of the external parts, until at last a powerful pain steadies the head, and effects its complete expulsion. At this moment (especially with a first child) the suffering of the woman is wrought to the highest pitch, and she occasionally experiences a smart rigor, or even becomes temporarily delirious.

After the expulsion of the head, there is commonly an interval varying from one minute to ten or fifteen; the pains then again recur, and by

* Vide Mechanism of Parturition, chap. 3.

them the face of the child, which at the moment
of expulsion, looked towards the anus, is turned
to one thigh of the mother, thus bringing the
shoulders into the long diameter of the vulva. By
the succeeding pains these latter are expelled, one
before the other, and finally the body and limbs
are driven out of the vagina, all being accomplished, in a natural case, by the unaided action of
the uterus.

It is not to be supposed that every natural
labour is divided exactly into the stages we have
laid down; on the contrary, there is an endless
variety of trifling circumstances. In many cases,
for example, the waters are discharged before the
os uteri is fully dilated; and again, the bag of
membranes may remain entire until both it and
the head within it are expelled from the vagina.
There are many variations, also, as to the length
of time and number of pains requisite for the
expulsion of the head, and subsequently of the
body and limbs. All these slighter differences
must be learned from actual attendance upon a
great number of labours; and when an acquaintance with them is acquired, it constitutes a main
part of the unwritten although most valuable
knowledge of the practical accoucheur.

Third stage.—Immediately after the birth of
the child, the uterus, contracted to about the size
of a fœtal head, may be plainly felt through the

relaxed abdominal parietes. After a short interval, slight griping pains return, and the placenta, usually accompanied by some clots of blood, is expelled, passing through the rent in the membranes in such a manner as to invert the latter. Sometimes, one pain is sufficient to accomplish this process, and it occasionally is finished by the last pain of the second stage. This, however, is not usually the case, and according to the observations of Dr. John Clarke, which I believe to be tolerably correct, the average time for the expulsion of the after-birth is twenty-five minutes. Whether it be done in a space of time longer or shorter than this, it is always effected, *in a natural case*, solely by the action of the uterus. The third stage of labour being completed, the uterus descends into the pelvis, and can be felt there (through the abdominal walls) contracted to about the size of the closed fist.

CHAPTER IX.

DUTIES OF THE ACCOUCHEUR IN NATURAL LABOUR.

HAVING now described the physiological progress of a perfectly natural case of parturition, it will be well to consider the duties of the practitioner under such circumstances.

In the first place, then, it is always advisable to attend upon a patient as soon as possible after being sent for; we can never depend upon the account given by the attendants, and should always satisfy ourselves as to the progress of the labour, that no opportunity for giving assistance (if such should be needed) may be suffered to escape. The only matters necessary to be taken to a patient's house are a catheter, a lancet, and a little tincture of opium; these may be suddenly required, and it will be well to have them at hand, but all other ob-stetric apparatus I would strongly advise to be left in the practitioner's study; if accidentally seen in the lying-in chamber, they cannot fail to excite alarm, and I think we should never familiarise our own minds to the idea of their being *ordinarily* necessary in practice.

In approaching the patient, some little tact is requisite; we should always first let her be apprised of our approach, as the unexpected appearance of a medical man has been known to affect the nervous system of a timid woman so powerfully as to cause a suspension of uterine action. We should, also, before seeing the patient, make enquiries from the nurse as to the period when labour commenced, the nature of the pains, whether there has been any discharge from the vagina, whether her bowels have been opened, or she has passed urine freely. Having ascertained these particulars, we may then visit the patient, and enquire from herself, how long she has been suffering pain? what is the situation of her pains? how often they occur? &c. We may also examine her tongue and pulse, and if she be in bed, it will be well to place the hand upon her abdomen, in order to learn if it has subsided, and if the uterus be disposed to contract firmly upon its contents. All this should be done seriously, but at the same time cheerfully, and without embarrassment or unnecessary assumption of solemnity. If the woman has had children before, and the symptoms show decidedly that she is in labour, we should not leave her without making an examination; but if it be a first case, and the

labour only commencing, there will be no necessity for doing so at once.

Young practitioners often feel a difficulty in first
proposing an examination : but the fact is, that
any embarrassment that may arise is generally
altogether of their own creation. The woman's
delicacy never should be aroused by any comments
upon 'the disagreeable duty that is necessary to
be performed,' &c. &c.; the thing should be done
(without talking about it) as coolly as if we were
merely feeling her pulse, and our manner should
never betray any consciousness of the operation
being in the slightest degree indelicate. If we
adopt this plan, we shall seldom fail in getting an
examination whenever we think it necessary; and
the only intimation we need make of our purpose is,
to desire the patient to lie in the proper position,
or to ask the nurse for a napkin, either of which
expressions will be perfectly well understood, and
we shall, in all probability, have no further
trouble.

Before adverting to the mode of examination, we
may describe the position in which the woman is
usually placed while it is being made. This is generally the same as that in which she is to be delivered, or what is commonly called 'the obstetric
position,' and differs in different countries. In Great
Britain the woman is always placed upon her left
side, with her thighs flexed, and her hips brought

close to the right side of the bed; to prevent the latter from being wet, a dressed sheep-skin or thickly folded blanket is placed upon it, and covered with a doubled sheet, immediately under the patient's hips; after delivery, the sheet can be slipped away, so as to make the woman somewhat more comfortable without any injurious disturbance. This process is termed by nurses, 'guarding or preparing the bed.' On the Continent, the usual obstetric position is upon the back; and among the peasants of this country women are placed occasionally (but not always) upon their knees, both for examination and during labour.

The patient being properly placed, we stand at her back, and pass the right or left hand (whichever we think most convenient) under the bed-clothes, with as little delay as possible, up to the vulva, into the posterior extremity of which one or two fingers are to be introduced. If the os uteri be not very high, it will be sufficient to examine with the forefinger alone; but should the latter not be long enough, we shall be enabled to make a more satisfactory examination by passing, at the same time, the second finger. In either case, our object is to investigate accurately the condition of the os uteri, and the nature of the presentation within it.* In searching for the

* It will also be well to take the same opportunity for forming a general estimate as to the size and formation of the pelvis,

H

former, we must recollect that it is situated very much backwards towards the sacrum, and that frequently the cervix, thinly spread over the presenting part, will meet our finger very near the os externum, while the os tincæ lies considerably higher, and almost beyond our reach. Under such circumstances, I have sometimes been enabled to feel it, by making the nurse place her hand upon the patient's abdomen, and gently press down the uterus.

The sensation conveyed by the mouth of the womb varies very much in different cases. Very frequently, when labour has been going on for some time, we can pass our finger into it and feel its edge like a thin free membrane spread equally over the child's head; when this is the state of the part, it will probably become thicker as dilatation advances, which will be likely to go on rapidly and favourably. In other instances, the os tincæ feels from the commencement thick and rounded, and sometimes firm and hard, as if tumefied in consequence of inflammation. We should always make part of our examination during a pain, and if we then find that the opening is sensibly diminished while uterine action lasts, and more dilated afterwards, and especially if the membranes are protruded into it during

especially in first cases, where we have not the experience of former labours.

a pain, we may safely conclude that labour has set in.

As to the time that will be occupied by the first stage, we must draw our conclusions from the extent of dilatation, and also from the progress that may be made in that process between any two periods of examination: if the case be a first one (for example), the os tincæ only sufficiently open to admit our finger, and the effect of each pain very slight, we may expect that the first stage will occupy a considerable period; on the other hand, if the opening be as large as a half-crown piece, and is enlarged permanently after every contraction of the uterus, we may look for a speedier result. The relaxed and apparently dilatable condition of the os uteri, and of the vagina and external parts, will also lead us to hope for a quick labour; while the opposite conditions warrant a contrary conclusion. In women who have had many children, however, we may be very much deceived, and should be constantly upon our guard, as dilatation often occurs quite suddenly, without any previous indications from the state of the parts; it should therefore be a standing rule with accoucheurs to deliver no *positive* opinion as to the period when a labour will terminate.

Having made our observations respecting the progress of the case, we must next proceed to ascertain the presentation. This part of the examination should always be conducted during the absence of pain and consequent relaxation of the bag of waters, as we can then most readily feel what is contained in the cervix, and also run less risk of rupturing the membranes, an accident that should be carefully avoided. In natural labour, we can, under these circumstances, usually feel the head from the very commencement: we recognise it by its roundness and firmness; and also by the sutures and the posterior fontanelle, whenever we can distinguish the latter. Persons who have acquired a *tactus eruditus* from frequent practice, will be often able to ascertain the exact position of the head, with regard to the bones of the pelvis; but such nicety is not to be expected by the beginner, and, in fact, is little to be desired, as knowledge of this kind should have no influence upon our treatment, and is only to be looked upon as a matter of scientific curiosity.* In making an *early* examination, we shall be often enabled to feel the presentation, by having the uterus pressed down by a hand on the abdomen, in the way already mentioned.

Having satisfied ourselves that all is right, and that the labour is progressing, we may withdraw from the room of the patient; our presence there during the first stage is not needed, and, by operating as a restraint upon the woman, may

* Vide Mechanism of Parturition, chap. 3.

even be injurious. When there is any probability of the case terminating shortly, it is unnecessary to say that we should not leave the house ; and the young practitioner should constantly recollect that it is better for his reputation to give unprofitable attendance in many cases, than to run the risk of having one concluded during his absence.

During the dilating process, it is not necessary to confine the patient to bed : she may be allowed at her pleasure to sit up or walk about the room. If she be disposed to eat, she may get any light food, as gruel, or tea and dried toast, or even a little beef-tea : * nourishment of this description will keep the stomach healthfully employed, and will support the strength, but no cordials or stimulating food or drink should, on any account, be allowed.

Medical treatment is seldom required in a natural case : if the bowels have been confined, it will be useful, at the commencement, to administer an aperient,† or, if the labour has somewhat

---

* It is often advisable, when we have to deal with dyspeptic people, to give a little solid food, as slops are apt to produce derangement of the stomach, which, in its turn, becomes a frequent cause of irregular uterine action.

† Castor-oil answers very well for this purpose, if the woman's stomach will bear it ; or the following draught :—

℞ Pulveris Rhei, Sulphatis Potassæ, āā Ə j. ; Tincturæ Rhei,
ℨ j. ; Aquæ Cinnamomi, ℥ j. M. Fiat haustus.

For the enema we may use the following :—

℞ Decocti Hordei, lb. j. ; Olei Ricini, Muriatis Sodæ, āā ℥ j.
M. Fiat enema.

advanced, to clear out the rectum with an enema. The bladder should be carefully attended to throughout the whole labour, and the nurse cautioned to encourage the woman to empty it from time to time; if retention occurs, it must be relieved by the introduction of the catheter.

During the entire of the first stage, the duties of the accoucheur are rather passive than active; his object, in fact, should be rather to watch that nothing interrupts nature in her operations than to attempt giving her any assistance. When the second stage commences, a little more interference is warrantable, but still nature should be allowed to do as much of her own work as possible.

There are two main points to which our principal attention should be directed during the second stage: one of these is the preservation of the perineum, and the other the promotion of an effectual and permanent contraction of the uterus.

Occasionally, when women are delivered without *proper* assistance, considerable injury is done to the perineum while the head of the child is passing the vulva: a rent of more or less extent (sometimes passing into the rectum) may take place; or, in some rare instances, the head (without injuring the fourchette) may be driven through the perineum instead of the natural opening, constituting what has been termed ‘a circular

perforation.' When we consider the extreme
thinness to which the part is spread out, and the
distension which it suffers, we may rather be
surprised that accidents of the kind do not very
frequently happen : and, in fact, a slight tear (at
least of the mucous membrane) does occur in
almost every case of first labour. To lessen the
risk of this injury, which (if it amount to any
considerable extent) is one of the most miserable
that can befall a woman, the plan of 'supporting
the perineum' has been devised. To this duty
the accoucheur must attend as soon as the first
stage has terminated, and the head of the child
begins to press upon the external parts.*

The most convenient manner of performing it
is to sit at the right side of the bed, and, consequently, at the patient's back, and to apply the
palm of the right hand (covered with a towel)† flat
upon the perineum, the fingers then passing upon
each side of the vulva. The left hand may be
employed in preventing the woman from suddenly
withdrawing, which she is apt to do during the
suffering of a pain. The degree of pressure em-

---

* Beginners commonly fall into the error of supporting the
perineum too soon. If pressure be made before the time specified above, it may have the effect of heating and inflaming the
parts.

† This is a useful precaution, both for the sake of cleanliness,
and as it prevents the heat of the hand from drying up and
irritating the perineum.

ployed should be merely sufficient to give steady
and uniform support to the part, but should never
be so great as to retard the advance of the head.
The employment of such an amount of force as
would have the latter effect must of itself tend to
injure the perineum by pressing it against the
sharp edge which the posterior margin of the
frontal bone often presents when the parietal bones
are much compressed together. By gently keeping
up a proper degree of support, we can generally
prevent any serious mischief; and the distended
perineum at length slides uninjured over the child's
forehead and face. When this is accomplished,
the great danger is over; but still the sudden
passage of the shoulders may do harm, and it is
advisable to keep up the support until they are
expelled. After the head escapes, we must change
the position of our hand, and place it across the
perineum, with the radial edge applied close under
the child's chin.*

Several minutes often elapse before another
pain comes on; and during the interval we should
ascertain with the index finger of the left hand
whether the cord is twisted round the child's neck.
If it be, we must draw it cautiously out, and pass
it over the head; or if that be not possible, we
may open the loop, so as to allow the shoulders to

* At this period the practitioner will generally find it convenient to stand up, unless the bed be unusually low.

pass through it. After this has been done, we should pass the same finger into the mouth of the child, and remove any mucus or membrane that might obstruct the free admission of air. The irritation produced in the mouth by this process will often excite the infant to breathe while its body is yet in the uterus, and will thus much lessen the danger of suffocation incident to a delay in the completion of the delivery. No attempt should, under ordinary circumstances, ever be made to expedite the passage of any part of the child: all should be left to the efforts of the uterus, which, when so much progress has been gained, will very seldom indeed fail in accomplishing the whole operation. When the shoulders have escaped, we are then free from all anxiety with respect to the perineum, and may remove our right hand, and simply allow the head to rest upon its palm.

It now becomes necessary to attend to the other point of practice which has been mentioned; viz. to endeavour to ensure a full and permanent contraction of the uterus. For the accomplishment of this purpose, we know of no more powerful means than the employment of gentle friction and pressure over the organ, through the abdominal walls. Accordingly, as soon as the perineum is safe, the left hand should be placed upon the patient's abdomen under her clothes, and the

uterus followed down into the pelvis, as it contracts upon and expels the body and limbs of the
fœtus. In some cases, when the uterine action is
slow, slight friction on the abdomen will at once
bring on a pain, which otherwise might not return
for several minutes.

Next to ensuring a *perfect* contraction of the
uterine fibres, it is of the greatest importance to
maintain them *permanently* in that condition; and
this we shall best effect by keeping up gentle pressure, and allowing no interval for relaxation. In
order to answer this intention, as soon as it becomes
necessary for us to attend to the child, we should
cause the nurse to pass her hand over our own, in
such a manner as that, when ours is withdrawn
from the abdomen, she may be enabled to grasp
the uterus, and keep up as effective a pressure as
we have been employing. Upon no account should
this pressure be discontinued, until an equal support is given by the adjustment of the *binder* in
the way afterwards to be considered.

Our attention is next to be turned to the child,
which has now been entirely expelled, and is probably squalling and kicking lustily in the bed. If
it be so, we may at once separate it from the mother.
Before doing this, however, we must interrupt the
vascular connection between the two beings, by
tying a ligature (composed of six or eight house-
wife threads) tightly upon the cord, about two

inches from the child's abdomen. A similar knot
is then to be placed about two inches nearer to the
placenta, and the funis between the two may be
divided with a scissors. The whole of this operation should be conducted fairly within our view,
which may be done by drawing out the child a
little, without at all exposing the mother. But
even if exposure cannot be altogether avoided, the
rule that we should see the part which we cut still
remains absolute, as respect for its mother's delicacy would be a poor excuse to the child for the
loss of its penis or finger—accidents which have
been known to occur in an attempt to separate the
funis under the bed-clothes. After the division,
we should carefully wipe the blood from the cut
surface of the part of the cord attached to the
child, to ascertain that the vessels are properly
compressed, and that there is no danger of subsequent hemorrhage.

Should the child not have breathed perfectly
after birth, it is better to leave it attached to the
mother as long as the cord continues to pulsate, and
to endeavour to excite respiration by tickling the
mouth and fauces, and gently slapping and rubbing
the chest. If these means do not succeed, and
the placental circulation ceases, we must divide the
cord; and in this case, if the child's face be livid,
it is better not to put on a ligature in the first instance, but to allow a few drops of blood to flow,

which may possibly remove the state of asphyxia, into which the child has fallen. Other means for establishing respiration should also be adopted, which we shall consider at a future period.

The cord having been properly secured, the child may be given to an attendant; and the next step requiring the attention of the accoucheur is the putting on of the binder. This important part of the paraphernalia of the lying-in room should always be examined at the commencement of labour, that we may not be disappointed in its qualities when we come to need it. Those generally used consist of a piece of 'pillow-fustian,' or diaper, long enough to go round the woman's body, and broad enough to reach from the ribs to the trochanters. More elaborate contrivances, furnished with straps and buckles, to facilitate their application, are employed by some gentlemen.* When we are at a loss, a very good substitute for the common binder will be found in a long pillow-case or check apron. The mode of application is as follows :—without allowing the woman to move, we slip, with one of our hands, an end of the binder under her loins, next to her skin; this we pass gently on until it can be laid hold of by an

* A bandage of this kind has been recommended by Dr. T. Beatty, of this city, which answers the purpose very well. I should, however, rather feel disposed to have recourse to it two or three days after labour; and, in the first instance, prefer employing the common and more pliable strip of fustian.

assistant (or by our other hand), at the opposite side, when it can be spread out, and drawn downwards, until its lower edge is below the trochanters. The nurse should never be suffered to withdraw her hand from above the uterus until we are ready to fasten the binder; which we do with strong pins, beginning at the lower edge. The force with which we tighten it should be sufficient to give comfortable support; and it will not be of much consequence even if it be felt a little too tight at first, as it will slacken upon the expulsion of the placenta. By beginning to pin at the lower edge, and placing that below the trochanters, we prevent the binder from slackening by slipping upwards, as the tapering form of the hips would otherwise incline it to do.* When the binder has been properly adjusted, a soiled sheet may be pushed a short way under the hips, so as to prevent the woman from being annoyed by the wetness of the bed; and, having laid the divided cord upon this, we must patiently await the accomplishment of the third stage.

When the first two stages of a labour have been conducted in the manner already described, the result, in a very great majority of instances, will

---

* That extremity of the binder which has been passed under the woman (she still lying on her left side with her back towards the practitioner), should be pinned over the other, by which means we draw up the pendulous abdomen, and give it more perfect support.

be a speedy and safe separation of the placenta, without any further interference whatsoever. Sometimes, the pain which expelled the limbs of the child will, at the same time, drive the after-birth into the vagina. Generally, however, the uterus remains quiet for ten or fifteen minutes; after which the patient will, probably, experience a slight griping pain or two in the abdomen; and if we then pass our finger along the cord, we shall, most likely, be able to feel its insertion into the placenta, and ascertain that the latter is passing through the os uteri. We need not pull, or even stretch, the funis, as the contractions of the uterus will almost always effect the complete expulsion. But should this not take place, there appears to me to be, in such a case, nothing wrong in re-moving the secundines from the vagina, provided there be no appearance of such vascular excite-ment as might lead us to dread secondary hemor-rhage. In doing this, it is still unadvisable to extract by the cord, as we thereby bring against the opening the broadest surface of the placenta. On the other hand, we shall very much facilitate the operation if we hook one or two fingers on its edge, and then draw it sideways, and with a slow rotatory motion, through the os externum.*

---

* Immediately after the placenta has passed out, it is well to turn it round upon its own axis two or three times, as we thereby twist the membranes into a sort of rope, and so have

Should the case not proceed so quickly as we have supposed, and should half or three-quarters of an hour elapse without any action of the uterus, it will be well to stimulate it by a little moderate friction on the abdomen, and by tightening the binder, or, if necessary, placing a compress under it. As a general rule, I would say, that no attempt should ever be made to extract by pulling at the cord. By doing so, we always incur the risk of producing laceration of the funis or placenta, or inversion of the uterus, or even (according to the observations of Dr. Douglas)* of indirectly causing retention of the after-birth, by irritating the os uteri, and thus giving rise to the spasmodic contraction of the lower fibres of its body, which that gentleman conceives to constitute hour-glass contraction. We may merely put the cord gently on the stretch, which will, perhaps excite uterine action; but if this and the measures already mentioned fail, the case becomes one of retained placenta, and must be treated accordingly.

After the delivery has been entirely accomplished, it is always advisable to wait near the patient for at least half an hour; and we should,

a better chance of extracting them entire: if any part remains behind, it serves to collect clots of blood, which, in their turn, occasion after-pains. I always make it a rule to examine carefully the placenta and membranes after their expulsion, in order to satisfy myself that nothing has been left in the uterus.

* Med. Trans., v. 6.

on no account, leave her then if there be any disposition to hemorrhage, or even an unusual vascular excitement. Before taking our departure, we should always carefully ascertain, first, that the uterus is properly contracted, and the binder well adjusted; secondly, that the pulse is regular; and, thirdly, that there is no danger of hemorrhage from the child's funis.

CHAPTER X.

VARIETIES OF NATURAL LABOUR.

CERTAIN VARIATIONS occasionally occur in the circumstances of a natural labour, of which the three following require some additional consideration :—
1. When the head is expelled with the forehead toward the pubis, or what is technically called the fontanelle presentation ; 2. Face presentation ; and, 3. Descent of the hand or arm together with the head.

The first variety often eludes observation until the head is in the act of escaping from the vulva. We may discover it by the presenting part of the head not being so conical as when the vertex presents, and by its not so readily escaping under the arch of the pubis; by the direction of the sagittal suture; and by the facility with which we can feel the anterior fontanelle* near the symphysis pubis. By referring to what has been said in the chapter

---

. * The anterior fontanelle is distinguishable from the posterior by its lozenge shape, its greater size, and its four (instead of three) concurrent sutures.

upon the mechanism of parturition, it will be seen that this presentation will often occasion a tedious labour : in almost every case, however, nature will be sufficient to overcome the difficulties. Some eminent accoucheurs * have recommended an attempt to change the situation of the head during the first stage of labour; but the observations of Nägele, already quoted,† prove that nature, in a vast majority of instances, effects the change herself, and that we are not warranted in any interference by the average result of those cases that are actually *expelled* with the face forwards. All that is generally necessary is, a careful attention to the perineum, which incurs more than ordinary peril.

When the face presents, we shall also generally find the labour tedious, from the reasons already laid down.‡ A considerable difficulty often arises in the diagnosis of these cases: the marks are to be found in the features, the mouth, nose, eyes, &c.; but, when the face is much swollen, as it usually is, it is often by no means easy to recognise these. I have known the mouth to be mistaken for the anus, and the case thought to be a breech presentation. If we can feel the mouth, however, we always have the means of discriminating, by ascertaining the presence of the tongue.

---

* John Clarke, Smellie, Burns.   † Vide p. 25.
‡ Vide pp. 17, 26.

In the progress of the case, the chin is generally expelled first under the arch of the pubis, and nature usually accomplishes the business unassisted.   It is neither necessary nor warrantable to attempt any alteration of the child's position in a face case : all we have to attend to is, to obviate the effects of pressure upon the mother's bladder, which is said to be more liable to suffer than in vertex presentations ; and to avoid injuring the features by frequent and rude examinations.   The face is usually frightfully swollen and discoloured at the time of birth, but is restored to its natural condition in a much shorter time than we could at first expect.

The hand or arm occasionally descends with or before the head, and may cause delay and difficulty by the increase of bulk.   If the pelvis be narrow, a necessity for instrumental aid may even arise. When the complication is discovered before the head becomes jammed in the cavity, it is possible to prevent the descent of the arm, by holding it up during a pain, and allowing the head to descend before it; but any attempts of this kind should be made with extreme caution, as, in endeavouring to keep back the arm, we might be unfortunate enough to convert the case into one of shoulder presentation.

Among the slighter varieties of natural labour may be mentioned very early rupture of the membranes, without immediate accession of labour. I have known this to occur three weeks before delivery, and yet the latter to be good, and the child alive. A slight allusion to this circumstance has been already made.*

In the foregoing observations, I wish it to be understood as my opinion, that the existence of any of these varieties of labour should not of itself be considered as sufficient to justify instrumental interference. Such, however, may be required; but in administering it we must be entirely guided by considerations that will be subsequently adverted to.

* Vide p. 90.

CHAPTER XI.

DIFFICULT LABOUR.

STILL following the division of Denman, we shall include under this head ' every labour in which the head of the child presents, and which is protracted beyond twenty-four hours.' Like every other artificial definition, it will be presently seen that this does not perfectly apply to all cases, and that a labour, for example, which has not lasted twelve hours, will sometimes be more entitled to the character of difficult, than one which has lasted forty. As this class includes a great variety of cases, we shall subdivide it into three orders :— the first including those labours in which the time is protracted beyond twenty-four hours, but which, if properly managed, may be accomplished by nature; the second, those in which instrumental aid is required, but such as is compatible with the safety of both child and mother, viz., the forceps or vectis; and the third, those in which the difficulty is so great as to render it necessary either to

diminish artificially the bulk of the child, or to provide for it a passage larger than the natural one.*

Difficult labour of the first order may owe
its origin to one or more of a great number of
causes, which we shall consider as divided into two
classes :—

First, those which increase resistance to the
passage of the fœtus.

Secondly, those which lessen the force of the
expelling powers.

In any individual case, causes from both classes
may be combined.   The first includes—

a. Rigidity of the soft parts.— When speaking
of the various conditions assumed by the os uteri
during labour, it was mentioned that some were
much more favourable to dilatation than others ;
we also find the same to hold good with respect to
the vagina and vulva. In some instances, especially
of first pregnancy at a late period of life, we find
the external parts rigid and hot, and devoid of
their usual moisture ; occasionally so much so as
to make a common examination painful. When
this is the case, we shall probably find the os uteri
puffy and rigid, and very little disposed to dilate.

This condition will be produced by any cause
which will excite a febrile state of the woman's

---

* In this subdivision we have not followed Denman, who
makes four orders, and founds them upon the different *causes*
of difficulty.

system; and thus it sometimes follows bad management in a labour, that, if left to itself, would have proceeded happily. Thus, rupturing the membranes during the first stage will bring the hard head of the child into contact with the·mouth of the womb, instead of the soft accommodating wedge formed by the bag of waters, and will excite a state of local fever, that frequently interrupts dilatation, and occasions tedious labour. Stimulating food or drink, the room being too hot, the patient remaining constantly in bed, frequent examinations, &c., may all be followed by the same effect; which may also be produced by the fever consequent upon neglecting to evacuate the bladder or to remove costiveness. I think I have observed a similar indisposition to dilatation to depend upon a jamming of the anterior portion of the cervix between the head of the child and the symphysis pubis, in cases in which the os uteri was turned more than usually backwards and upwards towards the promontory of the sacrum.

The treatment of these cases must vary according to circumstances. In the first place, every thing likely to excite fever must be strictly avoided: the room must be kept cool and quiet; if the woman be disposed to speak, the conversation of her attendants should be cheerful; she should be encouraged to walk about occasionally, but not so much as to fatigue her, or to create any febrile excitement; the bladder should be carefully attended to, and, if necessary, the catheter introduced; if the bowels be confined, an aperient should be given, and, perhaps, an enema administered, as recommended in natural labour; she should have abundance of cooling drinks, as tea, whey, barley-water, lemonade, &c.; and if she takes any food, it should be of the lightest kind. Where there is much vascular excitement, with quick pulse, flushed face, and heat of skin, in a plethoric person, it is almost always advisable to abstract blood. The quantity must, of course, be regulated by circumstances; but, as a general rule, I would say let it be the minimum required.* I think I have observed considerable benefit to result in such cases as these from the employment of nauseating doses of tartar emetic, in conjunction with, or as a substitute for, bleeding; but there certainly are circumstances under which the latter cannot safely be dispensed with. Opium has been much recommended as a relaxant; but it is a medicine the effect of which in parturition we cannot accurately measure: it may totally suspend the pains, in place of expediting labour by its relaxing effects. Opiates should not be given when the bowels are confined; but when these have been opened, and the woman is teased with ineffectual pains, we may often procure for her some hours' sleep, and do

* Would that this rule were made absolute in medicine!

much good by the administration of a moderate
dose (say thirty drops) of laudanum. There is one
rule which is very little attended to in the administration of opium, yet it appears to me to be of
great importance : that is, when we want to produce the sedative effects of the drug, never to give
it except at those times when the patient is naturally disposed to rest. A dose of laudanum, for
example, that, at night, would produce quiet sleep,
would, if given in the morning, stimulate and
increase febrile action.

The plans just recommended, together with
patience, will generally remove any difficulty that
may arise from rigidity of the soft parts. Other
means, as fomentations, the introduction of tallow
into the vagina, application of belladonna to the
os uteri, injections of tobacco, the warm bath, &c.,
have been recommended ; but of their effects I
know nothing from experience, and, *à priori,* see
no reasons that can sanction their use.

b. Tumors and diseases of the soft parts.—The
hymen is sometimes preternaturally strong, and
has been found in existence at the time of parturition. There may also be cohesions of the labia,
either original, or the consequences of injuries.
Such obstructions generally yield to time and
patience; but cases are upon record in which it
was thought necessary to divide them by an incision ; and some are described that even required

a division of the cervix uteri in consequence of obliteration of its natural opening. Tumors of various kinds, and herniæ of the bladder or intestines, by projecting into the vagina, have occasionally interfered with the passage of the child : they are fortunately rare, and must be treated according to circumstances; if we can pass them above the head, labour may go on well. At other times we may perhaps open tumors if their contents be fluid, or we may be obliged to lessen the child's head. The only general rule that can be laid down is, to take such steps as may enable the birth to be accomplished with as little injury as possible to the mother.

c. Disproportion between the passage and the body to be propelled through it.—A slight degree of disproportion may exist and render a labour difficult, and yet nature be sufficient to accomplish the business. In such a case the head often bears great compression uninjured, and is expelled elongated to a most extraordinary degree. We should remember this, and not think of instruments as long as symptoms do not imperatively demand them. The disproportion may be caused by the small size of the pelvis, or stiffness of the coccygeal joint, or by unusual size or deformity of the fœtus.* The

---

* The body of a dead fœtus may be swollen by the air disengaged during putrefaction, and considerable difficulty be thus occasioned.

treatment must be very similar to that recommended for rigidity of the membranes; we must exercise our patience, and avoid every thing likely to excite fever. Where we can ascertain that there is a monstrous formation of the child, as, for instance, a hydrocephalic head, we may, of course, give assistance earlier than if we supposed the child to be alive: in such a case, puncturing the head, so as to evacuate the contained fluid, will probably expedite the labour much, and save the woman a great deal of pain and risk.

The class of causes which lessen the expelling force includes,—

a. Original inertness of the uterus.—This may depend upon weakness of constitution, produced by any cause, or upon a deficient irritability of the uterine fibres. It is said also to be sometimes occasioned by over distension of the uterus, or by extreme thickness of the membranes. We might expect that persons in the last stage of debilitating diseases would present examples of this want of action; but women in phthisis, fevers, &c., will frequently expel their children without any difficulty a few hours before death. There are no cases more' trying to the patience of the accoucheur than those of inertness of the uterus. In midwifery, however, patience is always a safe ally; and, by merely watching the woman, taking care that her strength is supported by light food, and avoiding all the *lædentia* already specified, we shall find that, although the labour may advance by very slow steps, yet in the end the uterine action will not often fail to be sufficient.

Aperients and enemata are particularly useful in this variety, often (especially the latter) exciting effective pains. Opium has been recommended in very large doses ; but, when given thus, I have known it to paralyse the uterus completely; and I should prefer using it merely in the way advised when speaking of rigidity of the membranes.

It is in these cases of inertness of the uterus that we most generally have favourable opportunities for the exhibition of *ergot of rye* ; and it may be well now to notice that drug.

The *secale cornutum* or *ergot* has been long known to exercise a powerful influence over the gravid uterus, and when taken in certain doses to cause contraction of that organ and the expulsion of its contents.

That it sometimes fails to produce its peculiar effect on the uterine fibres is quite true, but this is to be attributed not so much to its want of power in certain constitutions as to want of due care and precaution in selecting the medicine for use. The *secale cornutum* is a very delicate, perishable drug, and unless it be taken especial care of, it soon falls a prey to an insect that devours the interior of the grain. This mode of destruction is greatly favoured by exposure to damp, and hence if the ergot is not preserved in a warm situation and in well stoppered bottles it becomes very soon unfit for use. In such a condition it resembles damp turf mould, and that substance might as well be administered with a view to excite the uterus to contraction. The fresh active grain of ergot is nearly black on its surface, which is smooth and uniform, unpierced by holes (which when present indicate that the insect has begun its ravages); it breaks with a smooth fracture, and presents a surface resembling that of a broken almond. If it be reduced to fine powder it is of a greyish brown colour, and has a peculiar smell, not unlike that of new-mown hay. It should never be kept for use more than twelve months.

The mode in which I have been in the habit of administering *ergot* is, to infuse a drachm of the powder in a tea-cupful of boiling water for fifteen minutes, and then to give the half of the infusion, with the infused powder, adding a little milk. If this has no effect, it may be repeated in fifteen minutes; but I think it unadvisable and useless to give a third dose: if the two first produce no pains, another will not have a beneficial action.

The circumstances which contra-indicate the use of this drug should be accurately understood. It never should be given until the os uteri is completely dilated, nor when there is malformation of the pelvis, or rigidity of the soft parts. If used when the os uteri is undilated, its•effect would be similar to, and equally injurious with, too early rupture of the membranes : under the latter circumstances, it might cause lacerations of the uterus or of the other soft parts. It never should be given when there is any preternatural presentation that may require to be rectified, nor in convulsions, nor when there is any tendency to head symptoms. In the first case, by increasing the uterine action, it would of course increase the difficulties ; and in the two latter it would be unsafe, for reasons presently to be mentioned.*

* As a general rule it may be stated, that this medicine should not be given when there is a likelihood of delivery not being accomplished within two hours after its administration; for it has been found that the life of the child is often forfeited if a longer period is allowed to elapse. This pernicious effect upon the unborn child is attributable to two causes, first the kind of contraction induced in the fibres of the uterus, and next the directly poisonous agency of the drug. The uterine fibres are thrown into a state of permanent spasm by the ergot when a full and efficient dose has been taken: strong and forcing pains are produced and recur with frequency; but when the violence of them subsides, there is no complete relaxation of the walls of the uterus, such as usually takes place when ergot has not been given; the fibres remain in a contracted state, and thus must materially interfere with the due circulation of blood in the uterine sinuses, and of course must, *more or less,* cut off the supply of duly vitalized blood from the fœtus. In addition to this source of danger there is reason to believe that the ergot exercises a poisonous influence over the fœtus ; and if these two causes continue for two hours in operation, the result is very frequently a dead child. The ergot should, for this reason, not

On the other hand, if the passages be well prepared and dilated, the os uteri fully open, and the
head low down in the pelvis, with plenty of room,
in fact, nothing but the want of pains preventing
its expulsion, we may safely use ergot in the
manner above mentioned.

It may be supposed that greater success would
attend the employment of larger quantities of the
medicine; but I am fully persuaded that these
cannot be employed without exposing the patient
to considerable risk. In several instances I have
observed delirium to follow the exhibition of large
doses of ergot: it almost invariably depresses the
pulse; and I have known it to produce coma and
stertorous breathing without at all affecting the
uterus.* If it produce these effects, it is manifestly
improper when any head symptoms or tendency
to them exist.

The first notice paid to the secale cornutum was
attracted by its poisonous qualities; it having been
observed, when taken as an article of food, to
produce gangrene of the extremities, and death.
When given to animals, it acts similarly; and,
from two suspicious cases that came to my know-

be employed, unless there is good reason to hope that delivery
may be effected within this time, which seems to be the limit of
danger to the child; and if the time be overpassed, it becomes a
question whether means should not be adopted to complete the
birth.

* Perhaps even paralysing it.

ledge, in which it had been largely exhibited, and sloughing of the soft parts supervened (no instruments having been used), I am strongly disposed to adduce an additional ground for recommending its administration only in moderate doses.*

When inertness of the uterus depends upon its over distension, or upon extraordinary thickness of the membranes, the proper remedy will be to rupture these with the finger-nail, or a probe, introduced during a pain. I suspect that these are causes of rare occurrence; and, from what has been said respecting the evil consequences of too early evacuation of the waters, we should be very chary of interfering in this way.

b. Affections of the mind, as fear, anger, &c., powerfully affect some individuals, and often so much so, as to cause a complete suspension of pains. Knowledge of this fact furnishes, of course, a strong inducement to keep a patient tranquil and, as far as possible, free from all mental annoyance.

c. Shortness of the funis is said sometimes to retard labour, especially when it is at the same time twisted round the child's neck. Such extreme shortness is of very rare occurrence. It might possibly be necessary, after the birth of the head, to tie and divide the funis; but such an operation ought not to be lightly undertaken, and will very seldom, indeed, be required.

* Vide Report of Wellesley Female Institution, in Dublin Med. Journ., vol. v.

CHAPTER XII.*

ON OBSTETRIC OPERATIONS—THE FORCEPS.

WE have next to consider the second order of difficult labours. This includes all cases of protracted or tedious parturition in which the presentation is natural, but in which (the natural efforts failing to accomplish delivery) it becomes necessary to have recourse to instrumental assistance of a kind compatible with the safety of both mother and child.

The chief aim of the art of midwifery has been defined to be 'the safe delivery of a living child from a living mother.' There can, therefore, be no chapter in a manual of midwifery of greater practical interest than that which treats of the method of accomplishing safe parturition in cases which must terminate unfavourably to either the mother or the child if nature be not assisted by art.

* The following chapter has been completely re-written for this edition, and the present editor is responsible for the opinions and statements it contains, some of which were first published in his 'Lectures on the Forceps in Midwifery Practice.'

K

In this country there are but two instrumental
operations employed for this purpose—namely,
the applications of the vectis and of the forceps.
The former is now so seldom resorted to that we
shall confine ourselves in this chapter to the
latter.

There has, I think, been hardly any improvement in the modern practice of medicine or surgery greater than that which has recently taken
place in the practice of midwifery from the more
frequent and timely employment of the forceps
in those cases which require its application.

I should be very reluctant, however, to advo-
cate, as some writers have done, the habitual use
of instruments in ordinary cases. 'Meddlesome
widwifery is bad,' as was justly observed by Dr.
Blundell; and it is obvious that the course of
natural labour should never be interfered with
except for the purpose of rescuing either the parturient woman or the child from danger, or for
the purpose of saving the woman from the sufferings of over-protracted labour.

Some years ago the forceps was seldom resorted
to until the parturient woman, worn out by the
protracted suffering she had endured, was all but
moribund; and when, too, the child was probably
dead in consequence of the long-continued pressure it had been subjected to. Thus, in the
hospital with which I am connected, during the

Mastership of Dr. Clarke, from 1787 to 1793, the forceps was only used fourteen times in 10,387 deliveries. In Dr. Labatt's Mastership, from 1815 to 1821, during which time there were 21,867 births, the forceps was not once applied. In Dr. Collins' time, from 1826 to 1833, the forceps was employed but twenty-four times in 16,654 cases. Thus, in these 48,908 deliveries, which took place in the hospital, and which were conducted under the rules then in force, we find that the forceps was applied only thirty-eight times, or about once in 1,300 cases. How different is this from the modern practice of the Dublin Hospital, in which, under the present Master, Dr. George Johnston, in the year ending November 5, 1869, the forceps was applied eighty-one times in 1,159 cases of labour which occurred in the institution. And in the year ending November 5, 1870, the forceps was used eighty-three times in 1,087 deliveries.

In private practice until of late years the forceps was even less frequently used than it was in the hospital. Thus, Dr. Clarke, in his private practice in Dublin, extending over a period of forty years, during which time he attended 3,878 cases of labour, only once attempted to apply the forceps and then did not succeed. Dr. Davis (senior) says that in his opinion, it cannot be absolutely necessary to have recourse to the forceps or lever more than once in 300, or, at most, in 250 cases.   And Dr. Davis (junior), improving on this rule, only used the forceps seven times in 7,371 deliveries—that is, once in every 1,053 labours.

Dr. Churchill's statistics, published in the last edition of his 'Theory and Practice of Midwifery,' shows a great increase in the number of forceps operations in British practice within the last twenty-five years.   Thus, in the tables published in Dr. Churchill's 'Researches on Operative Midwifery,' in 1841, it is stated that in Great Britain out of 42,196 cases of labour, there were 120 forceps cases, or about one in 351 ; while in France the proportion was one in 162, and in Germany one in 153.   But in the same author's work, published in 1866, we learn that the proportion of forceps cases in British practice has risen to one in 171, while in France it is now one in 140, and in Germany one in 106.

The history of the introduction of the forceps into midwifery practice is a subject of great interest ; but is a topic, however, into which the practical nature of this work will not allow us to enter at any length.   It is sufficient for our purpose to know that none of the ancient Greek or Roman medical writers allude to the forceps as a means of delivering living children with ; but an instrument very similar to our modern forceps was found some years ago in the house of a mid-wife in the excavations at Pompeii. The Arabians appear to have been acquainted with this method of assisting Nature in cases of difficult labour, and Avicenna refers distinctly to the forceps for this purpose. The instrument, however, appears to have passed into disuse, and to have been completely forgotten by all writers and practitioners of midwifery from the time of Avicenna until that of Jacobus Rüeffe, who, in his work on 'Human Conception and Generation,' published at Zurich in 1554, speaks of a forceps without teeth—' forceps qua dentes eruuntur '—for the purpose of delivering living children with —' ut si possibile sit, id quod protrahendum est educat faciliter.' Nothing, however, seems to have come of Rüeffe's suggestion till the elder Chamberlen constructed and employed the forceps about the year 1647. These forceps were confined by the Chamberlen family to their own practice ; nor do they deserve much credit for an invention which they only employed for their own aggrandisement. No description of the forceps was given to the profession till Mr. Chapman, in 1773, published an account and engraving of Chamberlen's forceps, which he had received from another practitioner who had used them for several years previously. Thus it was to Chapman, and not to any of the Chamberlen family,

that the credit of introducing the midwifery forceps into practice is due.   Three forms of midwifery forceps were used by the Chamberlens,
and it is enough to say that they differ from the
short forceps now in use very little, excepting
the formation of the lock, which, in Chamberlen's
second forceps, is similar to that of the modern
French forceps, and the thickness and clumsiness
of the blades.

The most frequent cause of difficult parturition
is the protraction of the second stage of labour
by inertia of the uterus.   Experience has established the fact that delay in the first stage is of
comparatively little importance, whilst the second
stage of labour cannot be materially protracted
beyond its proper duration without increased
danger to the mother or child, or both.   The
most frequent cause of this is inertia of the uterus.
Thus, out of ninety-five cases in which I have
used the short forceps this measure was rendered
necessary by want of uterine action in sixty cases.

The os uteri must be fully dilated, or at least
dilatable, for some time before the forceps should
be applied.   Denman's rule was that 'the head
of the child should have rested for six hours as
low as the perineum before the forceps are applied.'   Dr. Gooch extended this period of suffering and danger for twelve hours, and Dr. Collins
did not think it right to interfere ' as long as the

head advanced ever so slowly unless the child be dead, or unless some urgent symptom presented itself.' Dr. Rambsbotham and other recent writers shorten this period of expectation to four hours in ordinary cases. The truth is, that no rule of this kind is of any practical value. One patient may suffer as much pain and risk from an hour's delay in the second stage of labour as another patient would in six or eight hours. Therefore, the only point to be considered in each case is the actual condition of the mother and child, and the particular circumstances that may render instrumental assistance necessary. The proper physiological duration of the second stage cannot be either materially shortened or materially prolonged with safety to mother or child.

The fact is unquestionable, that after very tedious labours the proportion of deaths from metritis, puerperal peritonitis, pyæmia, and other diseases to which women in childbed are liable, is greater than it is in cases where labour terminates within the natural period.

If the powerful uterine action of the second stage be allowed to continue too long unassisted in cases of difficult labour, a state of inertia may supervene, which may prove fatal when at last the necessary assistance is given, by resulting in uncontrollable post-partum hemorrhage, the consequence of the exhausted uterine contractility.

Rupture of the uterus is another, though fortunately comparatively rare, consequence of neglecting to afford timely assistance in the second stage of labour.

Nor are these the only results of the dread of all instrumental assistance in midwifery cases which still seems to influence some practitioners. Lacerations, contusions, inflammation, and slough-ing of the vesico-vaginal or recto-vaginal septa, or of both, are occasionally the sequence of the long-protracted pressure of the child's head on the soft parts in cases of tedious labour.

The child's safety is as much endangered as the mother's by a very long-protracted second stage of labour. Not only is the foetal head unduly compressed in such cases, but also the body of the child, and especially the funis is exposed to the danger of a degree of pressure which may prove fatal if suffered to remain too long subject to the powerful expulsive efforts of the second stage after the rupture of the mem-branes. This consideration alone should make us at once interfere, under these circumstances, whenever we have reason to believe that the child's life would be endangered by further delay in the labour. It can need no argument to show that it is our imperative duty, when we have just reason to believe that the child's life is in danger, to interfere as soon as it is possible to do so, and thus to rescue the child from perishing in the womb, as well as to save the mother's life. The practitioner who under such circumstances would hesitate to deliver at once by the forceps would incur, as I believe, the same moral guilt that would rest on a man so devoid of humanity as to pass by without heed a drowning fellow-creature who might have been rescued from death by proper exertion.

A very slight degree of disproportion between the head of the child and the passage through which it has to pass during labour is sufficient to render parturition difficult. But in the majority of these cases the natural powers are able to overcome the difficulty thus created, the child's head being compressed and altered in form, often to a very remarkable extent, so as to accommodate itself to the size of the passage through which it is forced during labour.

Every student of midwifery who has any practical experience at the bedside of lying-in women must be fully aware of the extraordinary degree of pressure the fœtal head will bear so as to alter its form completely during a protracted labour without the least injury, and how rapidly it will recover its natural shape, often after a couple of days, from being elongated to an almost inconceivable degree becoming round again.

The compressing power of the forceps is gene-

rally supposed to be very limited, and the experiments of Baudeloque are generally quoted as
being conclusive on this point. This eminent
obstetrician performed nine experiments on the
heads of still-born children with Levret's forceps.
In one case the instrument bent in reducing the
head only two lines; in the next the sutures
were torn, and the brain escaped by compressing
the head three lines; in two cases in which the
sutures were loose, he reduced the head four
lines, and another case four lines and a-half; in
the seventh experiment three lines; and in the
eighth, two lines of space were gained.

These experiments, however, do not appear to
me to justify the opinion as to 'the limited
power of the forceps when used as a compressing
instrument,' which Dr. Murphy and other recent
writers join with Baudeloque in expressing. By
Baudeloque's own showing, he was able to compress the fœtal head as much as half an inch in
three out of nine cases, and, as was long since
pointed out by Dr. Rigby, the pressure which is
gradually employed by the forceps properly
applied to the head of the living child, the
plastic properties of which are so vast, will produce very different results from the violent and
sudden force applied by Baudeloque on inanimate
structures.

Disproportion between the mother's pelvis and

the fœtal head led to the use of the forceps in
several of my reported cases, the amount of disproportion being so slight in these instances that
the compressing power of the forceps was sufficient to overcome the difficulty. It should not
be rashly concluded that because a woman has a
slight degree of pelvic deformity, and because
her medical attendants in her previous labours
resorted to the perforator and crochet, that we
must abandon all hope of saving the child's life.
On the contrary, I published a case some time
ago of a patient whom I attended who had been
delivered in her two previous labours by the
perforator and crochet, there being some flatten-
ing of the curve of the sacrum, but who, notwithstanding this, then gave birth to a well-
formed living child by the natural efforts. Cases
have been recorded in which living children have
passed through a pelvis scarcely measuring three
inches, so that even a certain degree of pelvic
deformity may admit of the successful application of the forceps.

It may be a matter of much difficulty in such
cases to move the fœtal head with the forceps,
although perfectly adjusted. It may happen that
the accoucheur's efforts are thwarted by rigidity
of the soft parts, or that the child's head is not
yet sufficiently moulded and compressed by the
natural efforts ; in other words, that the forceps

is employed too soon, in which case, if the instrument be withdrawn for a time, we may again introduce it with perfect and facile success.

The forceps should be at once resorted to if from any cause during the second stage of labour the pulse rises above a hundred, if the abdomen becomes tender on pressure, if supra-pubic pain, premonitory of rupture of the uterus, occurs, or if symptoms of exhaustion or prostration, with excitement, manifest themselves. This instrument is also indicated in some cases of breech presentation, where there is peculiar difficulty in extracting the head, or if the sounds of the fœtal heart become weak, and if the cranial bones overlap much. It should also be employed in certain diseases of the heart and lungs, where danger may be apprehended from the protraction of the violent expulsive efforts of the second stage.

It is generally held by obstetric authorities that the forceps is intended only for cases in which the child is alive, and should never be employed to deliver dead children with. There is, however, one very important practical objection to this rule, viz., we can have no certain knowledge as to the child's condition until it is born, as all the means of diagnosis at our command, including the stethoscope, are very fallacious; and we would not, I think, be justified in relying so far on them as to do anything that prevents the chance of saving the child's life. I have more than once seen a living child delivered by the forceps in cases where no sound of the fœtal heart could be detected, even by most experienced auscultators, and where the cranial bones were loose and overlapping, and the discharges fœtid and discoloured.

So far we have considered those cases which are suitable for delivery with the short forceps, but there is another class of cases in which the short forceps is inapplicable, and which require the use of a longer and more powerful instrument.

The long forceps is intended for cases in which it becomes necessary to interfere before the head of the child has passed through the brim of the pelvis. These are chiefly cases of complex labour, such, for instance, as rupture of the uterus, hemorrhage in the first stage, puerperal convulsions, and some other cases in which immediate delivery is necessitated. The consideration of these cases, however, will be deferred until we come to speak of the varieties of complex labour. The long forceps is also required in cases of difficult labour where slight disproportion, or malposition, prevents the passage of the child's head through the brim of the pelvis—either to exert a slight degree of compression on the head sufficient to enable it to pass through the brim, or to rectify the malposition, as the case may be.

The midwifery forceps is a tractor, a compressor, and a lever of the first order, the fulcrum of each blade resting on the handle of the opposite side. There are two principal varieties of forceps, namely, the short and the long forceps. The former being generally employed in ordinary cases, I shall first describe the instrument which I prefer myself, and point out its mode of application. The measurements of this forceps are— ten inches in length from handle to point, the blades $6\frac{1}{2}$ inches long, the widest space between blades, when locked, $2\frac{7}{8}$ inches, the space between the points $1\frac{1}{4}$ inches. The total weight of the instrument is only $8\frac{1}{4}$ ounces, and a ring is introduced into the lock, into which the fingers of the operator is inserted during the extraction. The fenestra are very wide in proportion to the width of the blade, and so thin, that when the forceps is applied, the scalp over the parietal bones projects through in such a manner that there is comparatively little risk of the maternal structures being injured by the instrument.

It is a matter of great importance to apply the forceps properly, for although, in the hands of a dexterous accoucheur, and in proper cases, this instrument may be employed with perfect safety and facility, yet it must never be forgotten that in the hands of an unskilful practitioner, or in unsuitable cases, the forceps is a most dangerous implement, and its mal-use may produce effects as disastrous to the mother as to the child ; and hence we must now consider carefully the successive steps of the operation.

As a rule, instruments should not be used until a fair trial has been given to other measures. Therefore, in ordinary cases of difficult labour, change of position, friction over the uterus, and stimulating enemata of warm water and salt should be tried in the first instance. This rule we attach great importance to in the Rotunda Hospital, and very seldom resort to the forceps until stimulating enemata have been fairly tried, and have failed, previously.

Before the application of the forceps or any obstetric operation is decided on, a consultation should always be obtained, when possible. But if the medical attendant cannot procure the advice and assistance of another practitioner, he must proceed on his own responsibility, if the case be one that urgently requires instrumental aid. Before operating, the accoucheur must always inform the patient's husband or other near friend of what he is about to do, and if the patient herself be a resolute, sensible woman, he may also tell her that he is about to give her some assistance, but not otherwise.

The rectum having been emptied by the stimulating enemata already referred to, a dose of ergot should be administered immediately before putting the patient under the influence of chloroform, which is now generally, but not invariably, done in cases of operative midwifery.

The exact position of the head and state of the os uteri must be always ascertained by a vaginal examination immediately before the application of the forceps. I have more than once been sent for to apply the forceps in cases which the gentlemen in attendance believed to be suitable for instrumental assistance, but in which the os was found on examination undilated and undilatable, the cervix being so thin and tightly stretched over the fœtal head as to allow the sutures to be felt through it, and thus led the attendant into an error which, if acted on, might prove most disastrous.

The catheter should in every case be introduced before the forceps is applied. This must be done, even when we are assured by the nurse that the patient has passed plenty of water. I have several times been told so in cases where the bladder was so distended by accumulated urine, a little of which had dribbled away, and thus misled the nurse, that the progress of the labour was completely arrested by this cause, and in which it was only necessary to draw off the water to allow the head to come down without any further assistance. It is obvious how readily, if the forceps were used under such circumstances, rupture of the bladder might be produced.

The forceps may now be applied in the following manner. The patient being placed on her left side, with the shoulders drawn across the bed. and her hips projecting over its edge, the accoucheur, who sits facing the perineum, introduces the index and second fingers of his right hand into the vagina, behind the symphysis pubis, and passes them half round the circumference of the pelvis on the child's head, until he comes in contact with the ear, over which the forceps is generally placed. But whatever position the head may present in, the forceps should always, if possible, be placed in the oblique diameter of the pelvis, as if introduced antroposteriorly there is great danger of injuring the soft parts in the extraction of the head. The instrument being first warmed and smeared with lard, the upper blade is to be taken in the operator's left hand as lightly as he would hold a writing pen, and during an interval in the pains is to be gently and slowly insinuated between his fingers which rest over the ear and the child's head, until it has passed up so far that the lock lies at the fourchette. In the first stage of the operation the instrument should be passed upwards and backwards in the direction of the lower axis of the pelvis, but almost immediately it must be turned in the direction of the superior axis of the pelvis, and passed upwards and forwards.

The point of the forceps must be carefully kept in contact with the child's head to avoid injuring the soft parts, by raising the. handle gradually as the forceps slides over the convex head of the fœtus, excepting, however, as it passes over the ear, when it should be slightly depressed for a moment.

The handle of the blade already applied is then to be given to an assistant to retain *in. situ*, whilst the operator, now taking the other blade in his right hand, introduces two fingers of his left hand into the vagina, passes the second blade as he has the first between his fingers and the child's head, until the locking parts are in juxta-position, when, care being taken to prevent the soft parts from being caught, the forceps may be locked. If the handles come in perfect contact at their extremities as soon as this is done, it may be concluded that either the child's head is under the average size, or else that the instrument has not been properly applied. In either case very great caution will be required to prevent the instrument from slipping and lacerating the woman as soon as any traction is made with it.

If the blades have been properly introduced and applied to the head, there will be no difficulty in locking them. If there should be any difficulty, no time should be lost in striving to adjust them, but the blade last applied should be at once withdrawn and re-introduced in the right position.

When extracting the fœtal head with the forceps, the operator must bear in mind that the axis of the pelvis is a curved line; the axis of the inlet being downwards and backwards, and that of the outlet downwardsand forwards, and must make his traction to correspond with this. At first he pulls downwards and backwards, but as the head descends, alters the direction of his force till the vertex rests on the perineum, when he draws the head directly forwards through the arch of the pubis.

Delivery with the forceps should be as close an imitation of natural labour as possible. In natural labour the advance of the head is so gradual, that the progress effected by each pain is almost imperceptible, and therefore the forceps should be so gently used as to imitate in the slowness of its action the course which nature points out. No attempt at finishing a tedious labour by any sudden and forcible effort is justifiable ; nor should a desire to relieve his patient from suffering, or himself from a wearisome task, induce the practitioner to attempt by force what time, patience, and skill only can safely accomplish.

The rule of waiting for a pain before using traction with the forceps, and of acting in concert with the uterine expulsive efforts, is well founded, and should be acted on whenever the pains have not ceased before the application of the forceps.

To prevent the risk of lacerating the perineum, it is generally advisable, if there be sufficient uterine action, to unlock and remove the forceps when the occiput begins to emerge from the vulva, the posterior blade being the first to be withdrawn, and the head being forced out by pressing well over the coccyx and perineum during the pains.

After the head has descended into the pelvic cavity, the short forceps may be used in three different positions.

1st. Where the head is delayed at the outlet, the face lying in the hollow of the sacrum, the occiput under the arch of the pubis, and the sagittal suture lying over the perineum, the ordinary position at the end of the second stage of natural labour.

2nd. When the labour is delayed by the malposition of the head, the face being turned forwards towards the symphysis pubis, the occiput and vertex being opposed to the sacrum and perineum respectively.

3rd. Where the face lies to either side.

In the first position, delivery according to the rules already laid down is generally easy enough. In the second variety of position, the lock will be at the vertex and the point at the chin, and, by depressing this, the occiput will be drawn forwards from the perineum. The management of the third position demands no special mention.

The long forceps in use in the Dublin Lying-in Hospital is but a longer and stronger form of the short forceps already described, being sixteen inches in length instead of but ten or twelve, and is intended for those cases which have been pointed out, in which the head of the child is above the brim of the pelvis.

In England the double curved long forceps, recommended by Dr. Barnes, is generally employed. However, as this instrument is seldom used in this city—although I have occasionally resorted to it—I shall confine my observations to the straight instrument, which is not only more easily applied, but is moreover safer, although less powerful in its use. This long forceps is applied in exactly the same manner as the short forceps. The position of the blades must, however, be regulated by the diameter of the pelvis, and not, as in the case of the short forceps, by the position of the child's head. The long forceps should be introduced in the largest, or transverse, diameter of the pelvis, one blade being in each ilium, and when thus placed it becomes a matter of little importance whether they are applied over the occiput and face, or transversely over the child's head.

Forceps cases, like all cases of difficult labour, require to be very carefully watched during the period of convalescence after labour. As a rule— as the statistics of the Rotunda Hospital prove— forceps cases recover nearly as well as any others. But if premonitory symptoms of any form of metria or puerperal inflammation manifest themselves, it is all-important that these should have been looked for, and at once met with the appropriate treatment. The state of the urinary functions should also be carefully attended to for the first few days after all cases of difficult labour, and if there be any retention, the catheter must be used at least twice a day.

The vectis, or lever, is still employed by some practitioners, and therefore we may devote a few lines to the consideration of this instrument. The vectis appears to have been invented about the same time that the forceps was, and by some it is ascribed to the same inventor. By Chamberlen it was used as a simple lever of the first kind, the fulcrum being the pubes of the mother. The dangers of applying the vectis in this manner are obvious, as the soft parts between the vagina and pubes, namely the bladder and urethra, must be exposed to a most dangerous degree of pressure. Hence it is that, when resorted to at all, the vectis should be employed in the way first recommended by Dr. Dease of Dublin, about the year 1783, as an extractor, and not as a lever. The vectis generally used is a single blade of an ordinary short forceps. It is applied to the fœtal head in a similar manner to the forceps, and during the extractive efforts which are made with it great care must be taken to prevent its slipping from the head, or any pressure on, or laceration of, the soft parts. The vectis is intended for the same class of cases as the short forceps, but as the latter instrument may be more easily, effectually, and safely used, I prefer it to the former.

CHAPTER XIII.

PRETERNATURAL LABOUR.

THE TERM *preternatural* is applied when any part of the child, except the head, presents. The class has two orders:—1. Presentations of the breech, or inferior extremities; 2. Presentations of the shoulder, or superior extremities.

In the common parlance of the lying-in chamber, the term 'cross-birth' is applied to both these orders; but, technically and strictly, it is only used for the second, when the child actually lies transversely in the womb. Presentations of the back, abdomen, and sides, are described by authors; but if they ever occur, *at the full term of gestation*, the same principles apply to them as to cases of the second order.

Various signs of preternatural labour have been mentioned—as, peculiar motions of the child and shape of the mother; slow progress of the first stage; early rupture of the membranes, &c., but the only certain information upon the subject is to be obtained by examination *per vaginam*. In some cases, at the very commencement of labour,

we shall, even by this method, be unable to detect
any part of the child; and then, certainly, the pre-
sumption is, that the head is *not* presenting. It is
therefore incumbent upon us to watch the case
carefully, until, more progress having been made,
we may obtain the necessary information, and lose
no time in affording any assistance that may be
required.

The marks of the different presentations are as
follows:—*The head* is known from every other
part by its hardness, sutures, and fontanelles. *The
face* is distinguished from the breech by the forehead, by its features, and especially by the tongue.
Of these two presentations we have already spoken.
The nates are to be recognised by their globular
shape, softness, and elastic feel, by the cleft between the buttocks, the anus and parts of generation (especially in a male), and the free passage
of the meconium. In a first and hasty examination the finger may meet one of the trochanters,
when the part is pressed firmly into the pelvis,
and the skin tightly drawn over it; and I have
known it, under such circumstances, to be, for a
short time, mistaken for the head. *The shoulder*
is to be distinguished from the hip by its smaller
size, by the axilla and ribs, by the clavicle, scapula,
and by the arm, which is, in a marked degree,
smaller and more moveable than the thigh. *The
foot and hand* are to be distinguished from each

other by the greater thickness and length of the former, by the projection of the heel, by the shortness and evenness of the toes, and by the great toe not being, like the thumb, separable from the rest. The right hand can be distinguished from the left by grasping it as in the act of shaking hands, and observing whether the thumb does or does not correspond to the operator's. . *The elbow* can be known from the *knee* by its sharpness, and by the small size of the arm and forearm. All these things appear easy enough upon paper, or when we have a child quietly in its cradle ; but when it is in the uterus it is quite another affair, and tolerably-experienced practitioners are then not unfrequently at a loss. The way to prepare ourselves best against error is to improve our *tact*, by giving ourselves the habit of feeling the different parts of dead or living children whenever an opportunity offers ; and when we have occasion to exercise knowledge thus gained, we should proceed coolly and deliberately, without any affectation of extraordinary dexterity or greater skill than our brother practitioners.

Breech presentation.—The mechanism of parturition in these cases has been already fully explained.*   At the commencement of labour there may be two varieties :—1. With the front of the child directed towards the mother's spine; 2. With

* Vide p. 26.

the front directed towards the mother's abdomen:
the latter is considered the least favourable.

From the observations of Nägelè it is fully
established that, in a great majority of instances,
as the labour proceeds, the latter variety is converted by the pains (alone) into the former. More
rarely the child is expelled in the second position,
and then a degree of difficulty, requiring artificial
interference, occasionally occurs.

The first stage of a breech case must be conducted precisely as in a natural labour; the practitioner should be even more cautious than usual
in his examinations, lest the parts of generation
should suffer injury. If every thing goes on well,
nature, unassisted, should be allowed to expel the
breech and feet. If difficulty arises, it must be
treated according to the rules laid down in the
chapter upon difficult labour. The forceps or the
perforator, in short all the means there spoken of,
may, under certain circumstances, require to be employed. When the breech has descended to a certain
extent, if necessity for interference arises, we may
exert a powerful extractive purchase, by passing a
fillet (a common silk handkerchief answers very
well) over the groins, between the belly and thighs
of the fœtus, and extracting with it as we would
with a forceps.* A blunt hook is also sometimes

---

* The fillet can be readily passed by putting one end of it
through the eye of a long flexible probe.

used for the same purpose. When the body is expelled as far as the umbilicus, we should draw down the funis a little, so as to prevent it from being stretched. If it continues to pulsate, we may still leave everything to nature. Should there be any difficulty in the escape of the feet or arms, we may bring them down cautiously, taking care not to let them jerk out, so as to injure the perineum. To bring down the arms, we pass a forefinger successively into the bend of each elbow, and then sweep the forearm slowly over the breast.

In many instances, the expulsion of the head will quickly follow that of the body, the face turning into the hollow of the sacrum, as in natural labour. If it should not, and the cord ceases to pulsate, it becomes necessary to hasten the passage of the head, lest the child should be suffocated. The mode of doing this is to pass the fore and middle fingers of the right hand round the back of the child's neck, so as to give it a degree of support, and at the same time to place the forefinger of the left hand in its mouth, and depress the chin : by the latter manœuvre, we bring the head into the most favourable position for passing,* and at the same time, we perhaps make a channel along our finger, by which the air may have access to the child's mouth and chest. I have frequently known a child to breathe, with the greater part of its head

* Vide pp. 16, 27.

in the vagina. In general, by depressing the chin
we soon succeed in withdrawing the head,* but
sometimes a delay occurs, fatal to the child, and
it may even occasionally become necessary to perforate the head, after the body has escaped. The
perforator can, in such cases, be introduced behind
the ear. In all extractions of the head, the perineum requires to be carefully guarded. When
the belly of the child continues to be directed
forwards, up to the period of the head's passing,
some difficulty may arise from the chin hooking
upon the symphysis pubis. It then becomes
necessary to lay hold of the body of the child
(covering it with a napkin), and to give it a slight
inclination,† so as to bring the head into the
oblique diameter of the brim : the further steps
(depression of the chin, &c.), are to be conducted
in the ordinary manner.

Footling presentation.—This is to be conducted
precisely as the breech case, and is liable to the
same varieties. It is generally more fatal to the
child, in consequence of the slow, wedge-like dilatation produced by the limbs not permitting the
head to pass as quickly as when the large, bulky
breech has prepared the way for it. The funis is

---

* The extraction is often facilitated by pushing up the
occiput with the fingers of the right hand.

† In this manœuvre, we must recollect that it is very possible
to dislocate the child's neck, and we should therefore employ
force with suitable moderation.

consequently pressed upon injuriously, before the lungs can be supplied with air. The best way, in any case, to secure the speedy passage of the head, will be to allow the body to be expelled as slowly as possible, and even not to interfere with the head so long as the circulation through the cord continues. Efforts at disengaging the head should be made, if time permits, during a pain, but if the child be dying, we cannot, of course, wait for this.

$*$ In 839 labours which occurred in the Wellesley Female Institution, during the years 1832 and 1833, there were twenty presentations of the lower extremities, or one in forty-two. In both breech and footling cases, a considerable proportion of children are still-born.

Second order of preternatural labours.—In presentations of the shoulder or arm, the practice differs diametrically from that required in the first order : interference being in the one as universally demanded, as it is in the other universally forbidden. The mechanism of these cases, and of the 'spontaneous evolution,' by which nature occasionally relieves them, has been already explained,* but it is very generally agreed, that when the child is mature, we cannot safely trust to the occurrence of this natural operation, and that it is incumbent upon us, in every such case, to offer artificial

* Vide p. 28.

assistance. It is equally agreed upon that our interference should, if possible, consist in the introduction of the hand into the uterus, laying hold of the feet or legs, and bringing them into the vagina, in place of the arm or shoulder; in other words, turning the child. The circumstances of the case, however, may make a considerable difference in the facility, or even possibility of doing this, and may require variations in our mode of practice. The most favourable case is when we see the patient at, or are enabled to watch her until, the arrival of the exact moment when the os uteri is fully dilated, the membranes entire, or but lately broken, strong forcing pains not having yet commenced. If we are fortunate enough to find the patient in such a state, we should lose no time in turning.

The mode of performing the operation is as follows:—The woman is to be placed in the usual obstetric position, and the operator is to sit or kneel (as the height of the bed may render either posture most convenient) beside her. Either arm may be used: if we can ascertain* that the child's face is directed toward the mother's abdomen, the right hand will probably reach the feet more easily; if the face look backward, the left will then usually be more convenient. The choice of the arm, how-

* The direction of the child's face can be known by that of the palm of the hand and thumb, where these can be felt.

ever, must chiefly depend upon the operator's own
fancy ; but whichever is to be employed, it must be
completely bared* (the coat being taken off, and
shirt sleeve turned up), and well greased or soaped
in every part, except the palm of the hand, which
should be kept as dry as possible, that it may retain
a better power of grasping the child's limbs. These
preparations having been made, the fingers, collected into a conical form, are to be slowly and
gradually introduced into the vagina.   This stage
of the operation, until the broad part of the hand
has passed the os externum, occasions considerable
pain, and should be performed with great caution.
When the fingers reach the os uteri, they must be
passed in the same conical form into it, being
guided upon the child's arm, when it is down, or
otherwise upon the shoulder, to the front of its
body, where we may expect to find the feet.   In
doing this, of course we rupture the membranes,
should they still be entire; and our wrist then
plugging up the os tincæ, and preventing the
escape of the waters, we have, in the latter, a most
advantageous medium, wherein to move about our
hand, and seek for the feet.   In searching for
these, as in every step of the operation, we should

---

* We should not be satisfied with merely turning up the coat
sleeve, as we can never know beforehand how far it may be
necessary to pass up the arm.   The muscles also will be
cramped in their action by the tight girding of the turned up
sleeve.

be cool, and in no hurry, acting with our hand, systematically, and according to an imaginary picture of the child's position, upon which our mind should be intently fixed. If a pain comes on, we must cease, for the time, from moving our hand, and lay it flat upon the child's body, lest the projections of the knuckles should injure the uterus. If our arm becomes cramped, we may stop and rest for a little; a few minutes' delay making no difference in the success of the operation. When the feet or knees have been laid hold of we should carefully ascertain that there is no mistake,* and then withdraw them slowly, and with a wavy motion, out of the uterus. The subsequent treatment is precisely similar to that of a footling; some persons tie a garter upon the foot or feet as soon as they are brought down; but this is not of any importance, as there is little danger of their returning again. Dr. Breen, of Dublin, recommends the knees to be brought down in place of the feet, and they are certainly, in general, easier to be found. Other practitioners think it preferable only to bring down one foot, supposing the case to be thereby more assimilated to a breech presentation, and the chances of the child's being born alive to be increased accordingly.

---

* The second arm *might* be brought down in mistake for a leg; or, in twin cases, a leg of a second child. A little coolness will prevent either of these errors.

M

In another variety of the circumstances of preternatural labour, we may have the membranes
ruptured early without much dilatation of the os
uteri.   If there be at the same time no violent
forcing pains, we may wait a little, in the expectation of dilatation increasing.   Should the uterine
action be severe, means must be adopted for les-
sening it.   If the woman be plethoric, we may
bleed her ; should this not be successful or advisable, a very excellent plan is, to administer a
full dose of tincture of opium, say forty drops, and to
repeat it in half an hour, if the pains do not cease.
By either of these plans, or by a combination of
both, the contractions of the uterus will probably
be lessened, and relaxation produced, sufficient to
admit of the introduction of the hand.   It is
needless to say, that double caution is required in
turning, under these circumstances.

In certain unfortunate instances, we cannot by
our treatment stop the labour, or the fœtus has been
impacted into the pelvis before we see the patient,
or the latter may be deformed, and any of these
conditions may prevent us from attempting to turn.
We have then only the alternative of awaiting the
chance of spontaneous evolution, or of delivering the
child by perforation of its chest, and evisceration.
In depending upon the former, we must be guided
by the strength of the woman, and by the indications of the presentation, as to whether the process

is likely to take place or not; if we find the shoulder passing out and forwards upon the pubis, and the side gradually descending more and more, we may expect its occurrence. If it be not likely to take place naturally, evisceration will facilitate it, by admitting of a more easy doubling of the child's body. Some practitioners recommend in these cases separation of the head from the body, so as to admit of the extraction of the latter before the former; the other operation, however, is certainly the safest, usually answers very well, and is most generally adopted in this country.

Turning is seldom required before the eighth month of pregnancy, and never warrantable before the seventh: spontaneous evolution usually taking place easily, owing to the small size of the child. I have seen a living child born in this way about the sixth month of gestation.

₌ Four cases of presentations of the upper extremities occurred in the Wellesley Institution, during the years 1833 and 1834, being one in two hundred and ten. The child is very generally lost.

CHAPTER XIV.

ANOMALOUS LABOUR.—FIRST ORDER.— HEMORRHAGE.

In the class of anomalous labour are arranged a number of cases very dissimilar, and which, in fact, have no relation to each other, excepting that of not coming within any of the three former classes. We shall divide it into the following five orders :—

1. With hemorrhage.
2. —— convulsions.
3. —— plurality of children.
4. —— prolapsus of the funis.
5. —— rupture of the uterus or vagina.

1. *Hemorrhage* from the uterus, in connection with pregnancy, occurs under various circumstances : it may be considered as divided into four species :—

a. In early pregnancy, usually attended with abortion.

b. In advanced pregnancy, from the sixth month until the birth of the child.

c. Between the birth of the child and expulsion of the placenta.

d. After the expulsion of the placenta.

Before going into these particular species, it will be well to have definitely arranged in our minds the objects which we are to endeavour to attain in the treatment of every case of uterine hemorrhage. In the first place, then, we should have in view the general principle applicable to every form of hemorrhage, of tranquillising and keeping tranquil the excited circulation; secondly, we must look to the peculiar operation by which uterine bleeding is restrained, viz. contraction of the muscular fibres, and consequent compression of the bleeding vessels that pass between them. Upon these two principles our whole treatment in every case is to be based.

Abortion.—When the uterus discharges its contents before the end of the sixth month, we say that the woman aborts or miscarries; if the expulsion takes place after this period, but before the regular term, it is denominated premature labour. Miscarriage is always accompanied with more or less discharge of blood, and, as the latter is usually the most prominent and perilous symptom, the subject naturally falls under the head of hemorrhage. It is a very common accident, and occurs frequently in all ranks of life.*

The causes, of course, must be various : those which predispose to it are sometimes general or local plethora, but much more frequently general or local debility;† an unhealthy state of the uterine functions ; disease or death of the ovum ; and not uncommonly an obscure syphilitic taint in the constitution. In some women a kind of habit of abortion, at a particular period of gestation, seems to be established, which has been ingeniously explained by Madame Boivin, upon the supposition that in such cases the uterus has (in consequence of a former inflammation) contracted adhesions with the neighbouring parts, which prevent its enlarging beyond a certain limit. The exciting cause of miscarriage may be anything, corporeal or mental, which produces a sudden shock or disturbance in the system ; as external injuries, unusual exercise, displacement of the uterus, violent passions, severe cough, drastic purgatives, &c.

When a woman is about to abort, she generally feels, for some time previously, a sense of

* Among the women attended from the Wellesley Institution, at least one in eight has previously miscarried.

† Debility in these cases (whether general or local) must be understood as affecting specifically the generative organs, as the extreme weakness produced by lingering diseases (e.g. phthisis) is not usually followed by abortion.

weight and weakness in the loins and region of the uterus, followed by stitches of pain, shooting through the lower part of the abdomen, back, and thighs; occasionally there is frequent micturition and tenesmus.* Accompanying these symptoms, or immediately following them, there is always more or less discharge of blood from the vagina. This blood coagulates (thus differing from the menstrual secretion), and is often discharged suddenly, and in quantities so great as to reduce the woman to a state of extreme debility. When it occurs to any extent, we can seldom hope to prevent abortion; in fact, it cannot be of any considerable amount without an extensive separation of the ovum from the uterus, and consequent death of the former. Our prognosis, therefore, generally should be unfavourable, as to the chances of preventing a threatened abortion, although by judicious management we may sometimes succeed in doing so.

In some instances the ovum is discharged with very little pain, and in a short period; in others the process occupies some days, hemorrhage continuing more or less during the whole time, and not ceasing entirely until the ovum has been completely expelled. This latter fact makes us anxious to ascertain when complete expulsion has been

---

* Dr. Ramsbotham thinks *sudden* disappearance of the morning sickness a very certain forerunner of abortion.

effected, for which purpose we should have all the clots preserved and carefully examined. If we open them with a little attention, under water, the ovum will be recognised as a semitransparent membranous bag containing the fœtus floating in a clear fluid.* Parts of the ovum, as the decidua or embryo, will occasionally be expelled separately; and some mistake as to the former may arise from the resemblance frequently borne to it by a portion of the fibrine of coagulated blood.   When the abortion occurs at a very early period of gestation, the ovum is so small that our best directed attempts to discover it will often be in vain.

The treatment of abortions must be of three kinds.

1st. *Treatment for the prevention of a threatened miscarriage.*—In certain cases, the premonitory symptoms already enumerated exist sufficiently long and remarkably to admit of our interfering in time to prevent actual abortion. In other instances, the hemorrhage and discharge of the ovum are almost simultaneous with the lumbar pains, &c.   In the former case, our preventive remedies must depend a good deal upon the condition of the individual, and also upon the

---

* In very young ova the embryo is so gelatinous that it readily dissolves in the liquor amnii, and consequently cannot be seen.

nature of any constitutional symptoms which may exist. There is generally some degree of febrile excitement, and if it run high, with a quick bounding pulse, and severe pain, and the woman be plethoric and young, blood-letting is required, and will occasionally be of remarkable service.* The quantity to be drawn must entirely depend upon circumstances, and should be enough to produce a change in the symptoms. Generally accompanying a plethoric state we have evidence of gastric derangement; viz. constipation, nausea, foul tongue; sometimes there are headache and rigors. These symptoms indicate a necessity for purgatives, which should be of a saline and cooling description.†

In many forms of threatened abortion, where there are no symptoms of general plethora, but the patient suffers considerably from pains, we shall find great advantage from the employment of opium, when the bowels are free, or have been opened by an aperient. A full dose, in draught or pill, may be given at once, or five or six drops of laudanum may be prescribed every hour, in an ounce of infusion of roses; or, what is perhaps

---

* It is only under the circumstances above mentioned that blood-letting is admissible. I believe it to be, in general, much too freely employed in abortions.

† ℞ Infus. Rosarum, ℥viij.; Sulph. Magnesiæ, ℥j; Acid. Sulphuric. dil. ℨss. M. Sumatur uncia 3tia quâque horâ ad alvi solutionem.

better, a small opiate enema* may be administered. In general, I think, we shall find blood-letting less frequently called for than the latter plan. Under any circumstances, we must remember the principle of tranquillising the circulation, and accordingly should enjoin perfect rest in a horizontal posture ; a rigid avoidance of every thing stimulating ; a cool room ; cool drinks ; and light bed-clothes. In addition to these means, when there is any bleeding, we shall find advantage from the application to the vulva of cloths wrung out of cold water, or vinegar and water. By the measures just recommended, there is a fair chance afforded of preventing the accident, provided there has not already been much of the ovum separated. If this has happened, and is indicated by considerable bleeding, or we cannot prevent it from occurring, we must have recourse to the

Second line of treatment, for the purpose of bringing the patient with safety through the risks of abortion. The same general rules as to quietude, horizontal position, cooling aperients, &c. apply when we wish abortion to take place, as when we desire to prevent it. By some persons, ergot of rye is employed under these circumstances; but I cannot say I have ever observed any benefit to result from its use.

* ℞ Mucilaginis Amyli, ℥iv. ; Tinct. Opii, gt. xl. M. Fiat enema.

In many cases, the plan above recommended, if strictly persevered in, will be attended with happy results, and nothing more will be required; but should there be violent hemorrhage, and the assiduous application of cold cloths to the vulva and pubes * not be sufficient to check it, *plugging* must be resorted to.   This is an excellent remedy, especially in early-abortions, when the uterus is not large enough to admit of internal hemorrhage. It may be done with lint or a silk handkerchief, or (what, by entangling the blood, and promoting its coagulation, acts better than either) tow, or French wadding.   Any one of these materials is to be saturated with vinegar or cold water, and then passed gently into the vagina, so as to fill without stretching it.   A compress, wrung out of cold water, applied to the vulva outside, will keep the plug in its place, and in all probability the bleeding will be completely suppressed for the time.   The plug should never be left in the vagina longer than twelve hours, as the coagula are likely to become putrid.   Sometimes it will excite uterine action long before that period, and be ex-

---

* I must here interpose a caution with respect to the inordinate use of cold; where the woman is hot, and the circulation excited, it is an invaluable remedy, but its employment may be easily carried too far (especially in a weak person), and dangerous collapse produced by it.   The approach of this should always be attended to, when the cold applications must be removed and heat applied to the feet.

pelled, together with the ovum. When we have
occasion to remove the plug, if the flooding continues, a fresh one may be introduced. In its
use attention must be paid lest it should press
upon or interrupt the passage of the urethra.

Frequently the embryo comes away, leaving the
shell, or merely the placenta, in the womb; and
some of the severest hemorrhages I have seen in
abortions have been occasioned by a substance of
this kind preventing contraction, and keeping the
vessels open. In such a case ergot may be tried,
but I confess I have little expectation of benefit
from it. It is a standing rule never to attempt
introduction of the hand into the uterus before
the expiration of the sixth month of gestation, but
occasionally, by passing up a finger or two, we
shall detect the offending substance sticking in the
os tincæ, and be able to hook it away, when most
likely the bleeding will instantly cease. In some
instances, although there may be no loss of blood,
there is the most depressing sickness and nausea
occasioned by the distension of the os uteri in this
way, which will be completely and instantaneously
relieved by the manœuvre just referred to.

When the abortion is rather at an advanced
period of pregnancy, the placenta is often retained
for some days, in spite of all we can do to effect
its removal. It then occasionally becomes the
cause of putrid, fetid discharges, and I have known

it to produce low uterine fever and death. We shall sometimes succeed in bringing away the placenta when it is retained in this way, by the administration of a brisk purgative or enema : if the discharges become putrid, injections into the vagina of tepid water or infusion of chamomile *· must be frequently practised, and cleanliness very rigidly enforced.

The quantity of blood which women bear to lose in miscarriages is very remarkable. They rarely die from this cause, at all events before the end of the fifth month, although the prostration of strength is sometimes extreme.

Third line of treatment.—Practitioners are often consulted as to the means of preventing future abortions in those who have already repeatedly undergone them. The plan of treatment must, of course, vary very much in different cases. If possible, we should ascertain the cause or causes which operated upon former occasions, and remove them by suitable means. The great object is, to bring the patient into a good state of health—in the plethoric this must be done by evacuations, exercise, low diet, &c. — in the debilitated, by tonics, cold bathing or sponging, nutritious diet, good air, avoidance of all emotions, &c. In some individuals there is a disposition to abort at a par-

---

* Or perhaps injections containing chloride of lime may be found useful.

ticular period of gestation; and this may occasionally be passed over with safety, by keeping her for a short time before and after it in the horizontal posture, with perfect rest. The plan, however, must be adopted with caution, as the injury to the general health from confinement would in many cases be more prejudicial than allowing the patient to abort.

A very common cause of repeated abortions is a syphilitic taint in *either* parent. If this be ascertained, the treatment is obvious, but frequently its existence is very obscure. We very commonly meet with such a case as the following :—A man and woman, apparently both healthy, will marry, and the woman will abort, or prematurely produce dead children several times ; every variety of preventive treatment is probably tried, until at last a living child is born, which shortly after birth shows unequivocal signs of being syphilitic, and the case is thus cleared up: all this time, probably, the woman has never had a single venereal symptom, and the man not for years before his marriage. In some instances, there will be a succession of abortions, dead children, and syphilitic living ones. The remedy, under such circumstances, must be a steady, slow, mercurial course, adopted, I am of opinion, with both parents—certainly with the one known to have had the disease.

In managing a case of this peculiar description,

it is needless to say that the medical man has
occasion for all his prudence in order to avoid
being the promoter of family quarrels : the ascertaining of the history of the matter is particularly
difficult and delicate, and should be set about
with the greatest caution.

*Hemorrhage occurring from the end of the sixth
month until the time of birth.* This species is
always occasioned by a separation of a portion of
the placenta from the uterine surface, and consequently varies in quantity, according to the extent
of the disunion. It has two varieties.

1st. *Accidental hemorrhage,* when a casual rupture of the connecting vessels takes place, the placenta being in its natural situation, attached to the
fundus or sides of the uterus. This form may be
occasioned by blows, falls, over-exertion, &c.,* but
it sometimes occurs without any cause being evident. The whole or a part of the placenta may be
separated, and in some rare instances the centre
of the organ has been detached, and blood poured
out between it and the womb to a fatal extent,
while, the circumference remaining in connection,
no discharge or a very slight one has been permitted to escape out of the uterus. Accidental
hemorrhage may occur at any period of advanced
pregnancy ; if there be pains the discharge will be

* Dr. Ramsbotham believes that it is rarely attributable to
any apparent cause.

diminished, not increased, during uterine action, owing to the compression that is then exerted by the fibres upon the bleeding vessels.

As we are never sure that there may not be internal bleeding, our estimate of the danger to the patient must be entirely drawn from the effect produced upon her system. At this period of pregnancy the vessels are so very large that a comparatively small actual loss of blood will, from the suddenness of its discharge, produce more effect than a much greater loss during the early months.

If the hemorrhage be slight, our treatment may in the first instance be confined to those means, already specified,* which have for their object tranquillisation of the circulation. Should they not succeed, or the flooding be at first considerable, an examination must be made, to ascertain the state of the os uteri and the presentation. It is not advisable to be too forward in examining, unless the hemorrhage be of consequence, and actually going on, as otherwise we may only re produce it by disturbing the coagula, and the information required is often extremely difficult to be obtained by the finger during the seventh and eighth months, when the uterus has not yet

---

* Cold, horizontal posture, saline aperients, mineral acids, &c., vide p. 169. Blood-letting I believe is seldom or never proper at this period of pregnancy.

descended into the pelvis. Should the hemorrhage still continue, the further treatment must be conducted upon the principle of promoting contraction of the uterine fibres, and consequent constriction of the bleeding vessels. If we ascertain that the head or breech presents, it will generally suffice for this purpose to rupture the membranes with the finger nail or a probe, and allow of the escape of the waters. Pains will in most cases succeed this step, and effectually suppress the flooding : if they do not, or are weak, a dose or two of ergot and friction on the abdomen may be very useful in exciting or strengthening them.

In former times, the practice in accidental hemorrhage was, universally, to turn and deliver the child by the feet. Putting the hand into the uterus is, however, always to be avoided, if possible, and is not required, unless the uterus be absolutely inactive after the rupture of the membranes (a very rare case) ; or the presentation be a transverse one, which, on its own account, would justify the operation.

When labour proceeds, we must leave the case to nature, only paying double attention to the securing of a perfect contraction of the uterus after the child is born. Some gentlemen recommend the binder to be put on before delivery, but I prefer trusting to pressure by my own hand, which would be only impeded in its access to the abdomen by the employment of the binder at this period.

The *second variety,* or *unavoidable hemorrhage,* is so called from the circumstance of the placenta being unnaturally situated over the os uteri, whereby a laceration of its vessels and consequent bleeding is unavoidable whenever this opening comes to be dilated. The centre of the organ or a portion of its circumference may be attached to the os tincæ. In this form, the bleeding generally first occurs during the sixth or seventh months, at the period when the cervix is beginning to be developed ; and may recur at intervals, yielding, from time to time, to the adoption of general measures. When labour arrives, however (and often long before), a severe and dangerous flooding *must* take place, calling for the promptest assistance from art.

The unavoidable hemorrhage is to be distinguished from the accidental by the discharge being increased during a pain, in consequence of the dilatation of the os uteri rupturing additional vessels, while, on the contrary, in the other, it is at the same period diminished, owing to the pressure then exerted upon the already open vessels. We should always, however, satisfy ourselves by vaginal examination that the placenta actually presents. It is to be known by its peculiar feel, and I know of no better way of instructing a

student in this than to direct him to give himself
the custom of handling every placenta which may
come within his reach. By doing so he will in a
short time acquire a tact which it would be hopeless to attempt conveying by words.

The principle of treatment in a complete placental presentation decidedly is, to effect a total
separation of the organ, by delivering the woman
as soon as practicable. Whenever, therefore, we
ascertain a case to be of this nature, we must
carefully watch it, and seize upon the proper time
for artificial interference; that is, when the os
uteri is so far dilated or dilatable as to allow of
our passing up our hand, turning the child, and
delivering by the feet. If the hemorrhage has
commenced long before the period of labour, we
shall probably have to wait some time before this
state is arrived at—and a most anxious and harass-
ing waiting it is. The patient must be closely
watched, the ordinary hemorrhagic remedies employed, and, if these do not succeed, plugging
adopted. I think I have seen the latter measure
do excellent service, restraining the flooding most
effectually, and exciting the os uteri to a speedy
dilatation. The objection to it is, that there may
possibly be internal hemorrhage during its use,
but, if the vagina be well filled, this does not
appear very likely to take place, as the placenta
itself, when covering the whole os uteri, forms an

excellent plug upon that side. At all events, when the plug is employed, the closest attention must be paid to any effects that the bleeding may produce upon the constitution, whereby we shall obtain timely notice of any internal loss. If the woman retains her strength, we may wait until some dilatation takes place, but should she be weak, it is our duty to attempt the operation before she sinks, as soon as we consider the parts to be sufficiently *relaxed*, even though they may not be dilated. When there has been much bleeding, the probability is that the parts will not afford a firm resistance, and the case is always one requiring prompt aid.

In performing the operation, we introduce the hand, as slowly as we please, in the manner and with the precautions already laid down,* until it reaches the os uteri; it must then either be passed through the placenta, or by the side of it, into the cavity. During this step, the operator has need of all his coolness and resolution. There is usually a frightful increase of hemorrhage, the blood gushing in torrents along his arm; if, panic-stricken, he withdraws for a moment, the woman is inevitably lost; but by pushing on boldly and steadily, he soon brings his wrist and arm, as an effectual plug, into the mouth of the womb, and the discharge imme-

* Vide p. 159.

diately ceases. There is then time for consideration, and the feet must be deliberately sought for and brought down in the usual way into the vagina. There will seldom be any more hemorrhage, and the rest of the delivery is to be accomplished as in a footling case. The placenta will generally be found loose in the vagina: I have sometimes found it to come along with my hand and the child's feet out of the vulva. Great attention is necessary to secure subsequent contraction of the uterus, and if the woman require it, she should be supported with stimulants * during the operation.

Where there is merely an edge of the placenta attached over the os uteri, it will often not be necessary to turn. If we can ascertain that the head presents above it, rupturing the membranes may bring the former down so as to press upon the bleeding vessels, and there may be no further danger. It is often difficult to decide which step should be taken ; it is certainly very desirable to avoid introduction of the hand into the uterus, but where any doubt as to the practice exists, it appears to me to be preferable to turn. In some cases I have known the placenta to be expelled completely out of the vagina before the child, which, being driven by strong pains into the os uteri, effectually restrained the bleeding. In one case I saw a placenta completely separated and

---

* One of the very best of these is burnt brandy.

driven out of the uterus into the vagina, at the posterior part of which it remained until the child was expelled past it. Such cases as these, however, are mere exceptions, and afford no data for the establishment of any particular line of practice.

₊ The average of placenta presentations in the Wellesley Institution, during the years 1832 and 1833, was one in 167. The child is very frequently lost, and very great care is required to save the mother, especially when she has lost much blood. Dr. Merriman thinks that phlegmasia dolens is a common sequela.

c. Hemorrhage occurring between the birth of the child and expulsion of the placenta.—The surest means of preventing this accident will be, to follow rigidly the directions given in the chapter upon natural labour for the management of the latter stages of the process. The great secret is, to promote and keep up permanently a full contraction of the uterus : if we can succeed in doing this, we shall seldom have to treat either hemorrhage or retained placenta.

The manner in which this form occurs is various. In some women, in whom will generally be found an excited state of the circulation towards the close of labour, flooding sets in immediately

after the birth of the child, and by one immense
gush quickly produces syncope. In others, a slow
draining continues from the same period, until a
similar effect, or alarming prostration of strength,
ensues. Again, in a third case, the uterus contracts very well, and continues contracted for some
time, when it relaxes, and flooding takes place
with more or less violence.

In all these cases, the two principles already
laid down must guide our conduct; friction and
pressure must be made over the uterus, to excite
its contraction, and the circulation must be quieted
by throwing off the bed-clothes (excepting a light
sheet), removing the pillow from beneath the
woman's head, so as to lay her perfectly horizontal,
and opening the window, to admit fresh air and
cool the apartment. Cold cloths may be applied
to the vulva and pubes, with a view of answering
both intentions, cold quieting the circulation and
being a powerful stimulant to the uterine fibres.
When sent for to a case of hemorrhage, I have
often succeeded in procuring immediate uterine
contraction, by placing my hand (cold from having
been in the open air) upon the abdomen, which
the attendant (heated by his anxiety) had been in
vain pressing upon with all his force. Where
simple application of cold does not succeed, accompanying it by a shock, as by pouring a jug of water
from some height upon the lower part of the ab-

domen, will often be very beneficial. Introduction of ice into the vagina has been recommended by some; but where are we to get ice quickly enough to be of use in a case of violent flooding?* Should these plans not succeed in checking the discharge, we must, as a *dernier resort,* introduce our hand into the uterus, both for the purpose of stimulating it to action, and to remove the placenta, which, being partially or entirely detached, may prevent contraction and keep the vessels open. The further management of this variety of hemorrhage we shall consider in the course of our remarks upon retention of the placenta, which, from the close connection of the two subjects, may be introduced here.

Retention of the placenta may be occasioned by three causes :—1. Want of contraction in the uterus; 2. Irregular action of the fibres, producing hour-glass contraction; and, 3. Morbid adhesion of the organ to the uterus.

If the labour be conducted in the way recommended in the foregoing pages, the first two causes will very seldom exist. The first very generally arises from interference in hastening the birth of the child's body, whereby the stimulus is withdrawn too soon from the uterus, and it is left empty and without anything to excite its contrac-

* As has been before observed, we must beware of going too far with the employment of cold.

tion.   The same effect often follows, when the
womb itself expels its contents too rapidly.   On
the other hand, when a labour has been very
tedious, the uterine fibres are fatigued, and require rest for some time before they again act.
Irregular contraction is generally occasioned by
injudicious attempts at extraction by the funis,
which, without producing the desired effect, irritate the fibres of the cervix and excite them to
contract spasmodically, thus imprisoning the placenta.   This condition is termed hour-glass contraction, on account of the chambers above and
below formed by the uterus and vagina and connected by the contracted cervix.   Morbid adhesion is an occurrence over the production of which
we have no control.

Under ordinary circumstances, we need not be
uneasy about a delay of an hour or two, in the
separation of the after-birth.   But if hemorrhage
should occur, or the retention continue longer than
we deem safe,* not yielding to the friction, &c.
already recommended, we must proceed to introduce the hand.   Before resorting to this measure,
we may try the *ergot*, which sometimes succeeds.
The introduction of the hand is to be conducted

---

* It is not easy to specify a precise amount of time, the lapse
of which warrants manual extraction.   I should be disposed to
say that two hours after the birth of the child would be quite
long enough to wait.

in the ordinary way,* moderate pressure being made upon the abdomen by an assistant while we are doing it, and the funis put upon the stretch by one hand, so as to serve as a guide for the other.

In many instances we shall find the placenta partly expelled from the uterus, but with a portion of its edge caught and firmly grasped by the os uteri : sometimes it lies within the cavity, quite separated. In either case it is likely that the mere irritation excited by the hand, will cause both itself and the placenta to be forcibly expelled. If the uterus be quite inactive, and flooding exists, we must not withdraw our hand until some action has been excited ; occasionally, it will be necessary to promote this, by moving the fingers in the cavity, or even by rubbing with the other hand, or employing an assistant to rub, strongly upon the abdomen. When there is morbid adhesion, the fingers must be spread out from the funis, towards the edge of the placenta, and insinuated between it and the uterus, so as to separate the one from the other; every caution must be used to ensure the *complete* removal of the mass. When there is hour-glass contraction, the spasm must be overcome, by introducing cautiously finger after finger into the constricted part, until the whole has been dilated so far as to allow of the removal of the

* Vide p. 159.

placenta. The length of time which this requires is often very great, and no one whose hand has not painfully experienced the power of the uterine fibres, could believe that so much resistance would be opposed. The average occurrence of retention is very small, if the latter part of the delivery of the child be conducted properly and without any unnecessary interference.

d. Hemorrhage occurring after expulsion of the placenta.—In some instances this is occasioned by the after-birth being removed too hastily, before the uterus is inclined to contract. In others, the uterus relaxes, probably after it has naturally and very quickly expelled the placenta. This form of flooding will be very generally prevented by avoiding the first mentioned cause; by preventing subsequent relaxation, by friction, the use of the binder, &c.; and by keeping the circulation quiet, after *every* labour, by the most strict enforcement of rest in the horizontal posture.

When it does unfortunately occur, notwithstanding our precautions, the principle upon which it is to be restrained is still the promoting of uterine contraction, which is to be effected by friction, pressure, cold, ergot of rye, &c.; or, if these do not succeed, introduction of the hand. Coagula may have collected in the uterus, keeping it open, and upon their removal by the hand, contraction may permanently ensue. This should be kept up by a very tight application of the binder, with a compress between it and the lower part of the abdomen.

In some cases, especially where the binder has not been well applied, hemorrhage may go on into the cavity of the womb, without a drop appearing externally. Under such circumstances, nothing may be known about the matter until the woman's lips are observed to be getting pale, her pulse weak and rapid, and she becomes restless, tossing her arms about, and complaining of want of light and air. The practitioner may have left her, and things have gone to this length before he can be recalled. When he lays his hand upon the abdomen, he will probably find sufficient cause for the symptoms, in the size which it has attained from the accumulation of blood in the uterus. Pressure may succeed in stimulating the uterus to contraction and expulsion of the coagula ; but if it does not do so immediately, we have no time to lose, and must instantly pass up the hand with a view of exciting action. When such dangerous prostration of strength as that described has taken place, it will be necessary to support the woman's strength by stimulants. Burnt bandy (or whisky) I have found to be the best that I have tried. A tea-spoonful of it, with from five to ten drops of laudanum, may be given every quarter or half hour, until the patient rallies. Of course the strictest rest must be enjoined, dangerous syncope, and even death, having been known to follow the mere raising of the head under such circumstances.

In every case of labour, if we have any special reason to expect post-partum hemorrhage, and in every case where a woman has previously borne a number of children, a full dose of ergot should be administered, as soon as the head begins to press on the perineum.

If hemorrhage continues after the means before spoken of have been tried—if firm pressure on the uterus, the external application of cold water, or cloths wrung out in iced water, to the vulva and over the pubis, fail to check the bleeding, we must inject cold water by the vaginal syringe, into the cavity of the uterus as long as the water injected returns tinged with blood. Great care must be taken, however, to avoid pumping air in place of water into the uterus, which might prove fatal.

Should this not soon stop the loss of blood, we must resort to the powerful styptic recommended by Dr. Barnes—namely, the solution of the perchloride of iron, which may be added to the water injected in the proportion of one part to four parts of water. This injection acts as a direct styptic to the bleeding vessels, and as a stimulant to excite uterine contraction.

In cases of severe hemorrhage the windows

should be thrown open, and air freely admitted to the patient. Her head should be lowered to the level of the body, and a warm jar may be put to the feet, if cold.

Opium was formerly recommended in all forms of hemorrhage connected with parturition. However, we do not use opium in the treatment of hemorrhage during or after labour, except in cases of great exhaustion from flooding, when full doses of opium offer the only means of arousing the flagging vital powers, and afford time for the employment of other measures : or, in doses of from twenty to thirty drops of the tincture, in the treatment of persistent draining from the uterus after labour.

When all other measures fail to arrest violent post-partum hemorrhage, which, if unchecked, must soon end fatally, transfusion must be resorted to.

The operation of transfusion, first successfully performed by Dr. Blundell in 1825, has recently been much improved and simplified by Dr. Robert McDonnell of Dublin, whose operation consists in the injection of a few ounces of *defibrinated* human blood into the venous system of the patient.

The blood to be transfused should be drawn from a large opening into a clean bowl. It must be briskly stirred with a clean glass rod, and when the fibrine begins to cling to the end of the rod, the blood must be strained through muslin into a second bowl which is immersed in a vessel of hot water, temperature 105°.

The defibrinated blood is now to be sucked up into a small glass bulb to which a tube and nozzle are adjusted, and a small spring forceps put on the tube to prevent the escape of the blood. A vein being opened in the patient's arm, the probe point of the silver nozzle is introduced into the vein, all air being first carefully expelled from the tube by removing the clip and allowing the blood to descend, and the blood allowed to flow in either by its own weight, or by atmospheric pressure. The operator, by placing his thumb on the upper orifice of the glass bulb, can at once control the flow of blood into the vein if he observe any bubble of air passing through the piece of glass tube, which he must watch constantly for this purpose. The great points to be attended are the perfect defibrinisation of the injected blood, and the avoidance of any air entering with it. If the patient's face or eyelids are observed to quiver during the operation, or if her respiration becomes embarrassed, it must be at once suspended, or death may result from embolism.

CHAPTER XV.

ANOMALOUS LABOUR.—SECOND ORDER.—
CONVULSIONS.

THIS is one of the most dangerous, although fortunately not a very common complication of parturition.   Convulsions may occur, either before
labour commences ; during its progress ; or after
it has been perfectly completed.   The attack is
sometimes preceded by premonitory symptoms,
indicating congestion within the cranium, as headache, vertigo, stupor, flushed face, numbness of
hand, arm, &c. ; at other times there is nothing
whatsoever to give notice of its approach.*   They
occur equally in first and in subsequent labours,
and are, according to my observations, particularly
dangerous and fatal in the latter.†

* I recollect once seeing a fatal case of convulsions, in which
the woman was seen three hours before the attack, and complained merely of pain in the epigastrium, without any head
symptom whatsoever.

† Perhaps some explanation of this may be found in the
supposition, that in first cases convulsions depend chiefly upon
sympathy of the nervous system with the *unusual* actions going

The symptoms of convulsions resemble very closely those of epilepsy; the face is shockingly contorted, either quite pale and leucophlegmatic, or livid and bloated; the muscles are violently convulsed, and sometimes become so rigid, that I have seen a woman placed upon her side during a paroxysm remain in that position without support; the tongue is protruded and often bitten in the spasmodic motions of the jaw, so that the saliva, which is blown in froth from the lips, becomes tinged with blood; there is sometimes a rattling in the throat, and generally a sharp hissing noise, produced by the rushing of the air, in breathing, through the frothy saliva. The patient is quite insensible, and when (after an indefinite period) the convulsion ceases, a deep sleep or rather coma succeeds, often with stertorous breathing, and continues for some time, when, if the paroxysm does not recur, she slowly recovers recollection, and complains of headache, and soreness in her limbs. The countenance is heavy and stupid, and the voice hoarse and altered. The pulse differs in different cases, being sometimes quick and strong, at others weak : before the fit it is often remarkably slow. As the disease increases, the return to sensibility between the fits becomes less marked, until at last there is no interval of consciousness.

on in the birth passages, while in subsequent labours they may more commonly have their cause in some *organic* disease.

o

Convulsion cases occur very much in groups at certain times, and Dr. Ramsbotham has observed that they are particularly frequent in hot sultry weather, before thunder-storms.

The pathology of this affection is not well understood: morbid anatomy has not hitherto thrown any certain light upon it. In some instances it appears to be a nervous affection, depending upon the dilatation of the birth passages, and combined with a state of plethora and unhealthy condition of the intestinal canal. In other cases, it is probably connected with organic disease of the brain.

From the state of the pathology, we may infer that the treatment is not well defined. That which, upon the whole, appears to have had the best success, is the depleting plan; but it certainly is not universally applicable. When the woman is plethoric and strong, with a quick and bounding, or a full, slow pulse, bleeding is unquestionably indicated, and from $\text{\small{3}}$xv. to $\text{\small{3}}$xxv. of blood should be drawn from the arm in a full stream: if this appears to be of service, and the blood is inflammatory, it may be repeated as long as it is evidently required; or the temporal artery may be opened. At the same time the head should be shaved, and a cold evaporating lotion or an ice cap applied to it. When the patient is not plethoric, but weak and rather hysterical, with a feeble, rapid pulse, the depleting system cannot be proceeded upon with so much confidence. Even then, probably, it will be well to try the effect of a small bleeding, and the appearance of the blood will be a good guide as to whether we should proceed. In a doubtful case, I should certainly be disposed to lean to the side of depletion. I have never seen a case of convulsions recover unless the bowels have been got to act, and then the secretions have been always depraved; therefore I think the use of purgative measures never should be omitted. A bolus of calomel and jalap* may be laid upon the tongue, and followed by a purgative mixture,† if we can get the patient to swallow. At the same time a purgative enema, containing an ounce of spirits of turpentine, may be thrown up. During the paroxysm Dr. Denman strongly recommends dashing the face with cold water, and it certainly often appears to shorten the fit. A solution of tartar emetic has lately been recommended, in nauseating doses, and I have sometimes thought that it produced good effects. Yet more recently chloroform has been employed, successfully, in combination with bleeding, apart from which, however, it is not to be relied upon; nor is its employment safe.

* ℞ Calomelanos, gr. v.; Pulv. Jalapæ, gr. x.; Conservæ Rosarum, q. s. ut fiat bolus.

† ℞ Inf. Sennæ, ℥vj.; Sulph. Magnesiæ, Tincturæ Jalapæ, āā ʒvj. M. Sumatur, ℥j. 2da quâque horâ ad effectum.

The foregoing plans apply to all varieties of puerperal convulsions; but when they occur before or during labour, a question arises as to whether or not the woman should be delivered. The solution of this question depends very much upon circumstances: if the woman be actually in labour, and sufficient advance made to admit of the application of the forceps, it will be generally advisable to deliver her; but I think no operation, neither turning nor perforation, ought to be attempted while the os uteri is rigid, and a risk exists of injuring it and thereby increasing irritation. Where all other means fail, and the case is evidently going to the bad, it may be better to perforate than to allow the patient to die undelivered; but I should feel the less encouraged to adopt this practice from the facts, that convulsions may get well, and the labour not come on for several hours, and even days, after; and again, that they may proceed to a fatal termination, even though delivery has taken place.*

By some persons it has been supposed that convulsions *always* depend upon mere *irritability* of the nervous system; and, in pursuance of their theory, they have universally treated the disease with opiates. As a general theory or practice, this

---

* I lately ruptured the membranes in a case of convulsions at the sixth month of pregnancy, after all other means had failed. Labour was completed in four hours after, but the woman did not recover.

is decidedly wrong; but I have already hinted at
a similar opinion with respect to bloodletting, and
it appears to me that, although a great number of
cases absolutely require the latter treatment, still
that some would succeed better under the former.
The two plans, also, may be used conjointly with
great benefit. Opium is indicated when the patient
is weak and debilitated, with a quick unsteady
pulse, and is naturally of an irritable temperament,
and when, if blood has been drawn, it is evidently
not inflammatory. After bleeding has been pre-
mised properly and beneficially, and the disease
begins to yield, an opiate will tranquillise the
system, and produce great benefit. The medicine
may be used in any convenient form. When the
patient can be got to swallow it, I should prefer
the Dover's powder, as likely to favour a useful
determination to the skin. The black drop answers
very well, as, from its small bulk, it can be laid
upon the tongue. The tincture of opium may be
conveniently given as an enema, should that mode
of administration be thought advisable. Should
the violence of the disease abate, which may be
known by an increase taking place in the length
of the interval, and a decrease in that of the fit,
we may of course diminish the energy of our treatment; still, however, continuing to act moderately
upon the same principle as at first, and adding, if
necessary, the application of blisters to the back

of the neck or head. During recovery, the use of the catheter will usually be required.

Convalescence is generally slow, and it is often a long time before the functions of the brain return to their healthy state, the disease sometimes even passing into mania. Very frequently the woman is quite insensible of all that has occurred during her illness, and I have known the failure of memory to be extended to a period of some days before the attack, when there *appeared* to be no morbid condition in existence.

₊ It is difficult to strike any average with respect to the relative frequency of convulsions. In the Wellesley Institution, during 1832, there was not a single case; while, in 1833, there were three—one before, one during, and one after delivery: the two latter recovered, the first was fatal.

Sudden death after delivery may be here briefly alluded to. It happens occasionally in the most unaccountable manner. A woman, for example, will go through her labour up to its perfect completion without any remarkable occurrence, and shortly afterwards, upon moving abruptly, raising her head to take a drink, or during the disturbance necessary to admit of her evacuating her ` bowels, she will be seized with sudden faintness, and immediately expire. More rarely the same event occurs some days after parturition.

The pathology of this occurrence is little known : it appears to be in some way connected with a sudden removal of pressure from the contents of the abdomen, and is often called 'a shock upon the nervous system;' a form of words which, I apprehend, is to be considered merely as conveying the negative information, that we cannot discover any organic lesion to which it may fairly be attributed. I once saw a woman die of apoplexy within twelve hours after a natural and good labour; she fell asleep a few minutes after delivery, and never awoke. On examination, several ounces of coagulated blood were found in the ventricles, and a large quantity of serum at the base of the brain.

Treatment in the former cases is almost unnecessary to be spoken of, as we seldom have time to employ any; if we meet an instance of dangerous syncope, we must exhibit stimulants, ammonia, ether, and, above all, burnt brandy, or mulled wine. Should the patient rally a little, light strengthening nourishment should be given in · small quantities, and all motion or active purgation avoided for several days.

The knowledge that such accidents now and then happen, should make us doubly attentive about several particulars in the treatment of lying-in women : for instance, with respect to the proper application of the binder, with a view (in reference to this subject) of supporting the abdominal viscera; also as to the observance of perfect rest and quietude, in a horizontal posture. The necessity for these attentions cannot be too strongly impressed upon the mind of the young practitioner.

CHAPTER XVI.

ANOMALOUS LABOUR.—THIRD ORDER.— PLURALITY OF CHILDREN.

THE PROPORTION in which this variety of labour occurs, appears to vary very much in different places. For instance, in the Hospice de la Maternité of Paris, twins are stated by Madame Boivin to average about 1 in 132, and triplets 2 in 20,357; while, in the Dublin Lying-in Hospital, twins were found to occur as about 1 to 60, and triplets and quadruplets 1 to 4,300.*

Nothing can be certainly known as to the existence of a second or third child in the uterus, until the first is born, excepting in some few instances, where different parts of two children have been recognised, at the same time, in the vagina. It follows from this that the labour of the first should be conducted, in all respects, as it would under ordinary circumstances, interfering or not interfering, just as may be necessary, in accord-

* In the Wellesley Institution the proportion of twins has been about one in sixty-four.

ance with the rules for managing the various kinds of single labour, already laid down. When the first child is born, we at once know that there is another, when, in placing our left hand upon the abdomen, as has been already directed, we find that the uterus has very little diminished in size. An examination will then enable us to feel the membranes of the second child, and its presentation. Very commonly the uterus resumes its efforts in a few minutes, and, in consequence of the passages being well dilated, the second labour will go on very speedily, if there be nothing in the presentation to prevent it. Occasionally, however, there may be a delay of hours or even days between the two births, unless the latter be artificially hastened. It is not easy to lay down a rule as to when we should interfere, but there is no necessity for much haste unless some untoward circumstances arise.

After the first birth has been concluded, we may put on a binder, with moderate tightness, and when we have waited as long as (according to our judgment) is sufficient to allow the womb to recover from its fatigue,* it will be advisable to rupture the second membranes. After this step, should pains not return, a dose of *ergot* may be given, and we should not resort to the introduc-

* This period must vary, according to the circumstances of the first labour, strength, and spirit of the patient, &c.

tion of the hand in a natural case, until we ascertain that these means are ineffectual. Should the second child present transversely, it is better to introduce the hand, and turn at once; and the same advice holds good in case of any circumstance arising that might endanger the mother—as convulsions, hemorrhage, syncope, &c. Occasionally, the second child requires to be delivered with the forceps, in consequence of those symptoms presenting themselves, which, in an ordinary case, would lead us to the use of that instrument. When the first labour has been tedious and bad, or has required assistance, it will generally be prudent to expedite the second. In short, the rules to guide us in giving assistance in twin cases differ very little from those that ordinarily apply in single labour.

No attempt should ever be made to bring away the placenta, until both children have been delivered: as there is often but one for the two fœtuses, and even if there were two perfectly separate, removing the first, while a child remained in utero, would be leaving a bleeding surface with an uncontracted womb. The management of the after-births, subsequently, is to be conducted on the same principles as in single labour. When we have occasion to remove them, both should be taken away together, for the reason just now stated.

It is a general rule to keep the mother, as long as possible, ignorant of the existence of a second child, in order to prevent her from being dispirited, which might interfere with the further action of the uterus. All the rules appropriate to twin cases apply equally when there are three or more children in the womb. The more numerous the children, the more easy may parturition be expected to be, in consequence of their diminished size.

CHAPTER XVII.

ANOMALOUS LABOUR.—FOURTH ORDER.—
PRESENTATION OF THE FUNIS.

THIS ACCIDENT should rather be called prolapsus
of the funis, as it merely slips down past the presentation, whatever that may be. The peculiar
difficulties of the case refer entirely to the child,
whose life is placed in extreme peril, from the
probability of such pressure being exerted upon
the cord as will stop circulation through it long
before respiration can commence. There is no
danger to the mother, and consequently no ground
for interference, if, from the want of pulsation in
the funis, we ascertain that the child is already
dead, when we discover the nature of the case.
Should it be otherwise, we must endeavour to
obviate the injurious effects of pressure, which,
however, is not easy to be accomplished.

The most feasible plan is to endeavour to pass
up the cord above the presentation, and keep it
there during the pain, until the latter fills the
pelvis, and prevents it from again prolapsing.

Some have recommended to hook it upon a limb of the child, if possible: others to enclose it in a bag, or pass a sponge after it, to keep it up. Any of these means, that are likely to do no harm to the mother, should be tried; but I cannot say the same with respect to some instruments that have been contrived for returning the funis. The chance of our saving the child by their use is doubtful in the extreme; and, upon so slight a chance, no prudent man will run the risk of injuring the uterus, which must be more or less hazarded by the employment of those machines. Some gentlemen have spoken of delivering by turning or the forceps in funis presentations, but, I should hope, not seriously intending their suggestions to be adopted. It must be obvious to the most inexperienced, that the danger of pressure, in either of these operations, would be much greater than if the simple action of the uterus were trusted to.

₊ The proportion of funis presentations occurring in the Wellesley Institution, during the years 1832 and 1833, was 2 in 839.

CHAPTER XVIII.

ANOMALOUS LABOUR.—FIFTH ORDER.—RUPTURE
OF UTERUS OR VAGINA.

THIS is probably the most fatal complication of labour that can occur. It happens generally to individuals who have had a number of children, and in whom, consequently, the walls of the womb have been thinned and weakened by repeated distension. It is likely to occur when the pelvis is deformed, and, especially, when there is any sharp bony projection (*e. g.* a deformed sacral promontory), by pressure against which the uterus may be injured. The organ may also rupture itself upon the projecting limbs of the child, in a preternatural presentation, or it may be torn by the hand of the operator in turning.

The usual time for this accident to occur is in the course of a tedious labour, but it has happened when there was no unusual difficulty, and even, in some instances, long before the termination of pregnancy, so that it is very probable that, in most cases of rupture, there exists some previous disease of the uterus which renders it particularly liable to laceration.

The improper and violent use of the forceps has, I believe, much oftener than is supposed, produced laceration of the vagina.

When the accident happens during childbirth, the symptoms are generally very remarkable. A severe labour pain will, probably, suddenly cease, and the patient, at the same time, will be sensible of something giving way internally. The presentation, unless it be firmly locked in the pelvis, will then immediately be found to recede, often out of reach of the finger; at the same time the limbs may, perhaps, be felt through the parietes of the abdomen, and there will be some hemorrhage from the vagina. Great languor and prostration of strength soon follow, indicated by quick, weak, unsteady pulse, laboured respiration, and cold sweats. At the moment of the accident, the stomach will sometimes reject its contents, and shortly afterwards there will be vomiting of the brownish matter, so well known from its resemblance to coffee grounds: the pains entirely cease from the time of the rupture. The situation of the rupture is usually either transversely at the place where the cervix impinges upon the promontory of the sacrum, or where the cervix and vagina join, in which case both vagina and uterus are often involved in the rent; it may also happen at any part of the fundus.

The treatment generally adopted in these cases is to deliver the woman as soon as possible. If the head presents, and has not receded, this may be done with the forceps or perforator, whichever, from circumstances, may be considered most advisable. Should the child have partially escaped, through the rent, into the abdomen, the hand must be introduced, turning performed, and delivery accomplished by the feet. When the child has passed entirely out of the uterus, some practitioners recommend that delivery should not be attempted, but the further disposal of the foetus entrusted to nature, there being a remote probability of its being discharged, by an ulcerative process, through the abdominal walls. The choice left to us is a melancholy one, and I am not aware that much can be said in favour of either one plan or the other.

The subsequent treatment must be entirely guided by circumstances, and by the general medical and surgical knowledge of the practitioner. What is to be dreaded, is, first, the sinking and death of the patient, in a few hours, from the violence of the shock; and subsequently, if she rallies from this, peritoneal inflammation. Until some degree of reaction sets in, we shall probably find it necessary to give stimulants ; afterwards, we must treat the case according to the symptoms. The peritonitis is generally of a low kind,

P

accompanied with typhoid symptoms, and will seldom bear the free use of the lancet. Leeches to the abdomen, and opium in large doses, or calomel and opium, have, perhaps, more reasonable indications in their favour than any other plans. I should feel particularly disposed to avoid the use of any purgatives, excepting mild enemata.

The chances of the patient escaping are, of course, very slight ; but still instances of recovery have occurred, and we should not altogether despair as long as there is a spark of hope.

Laceration of an over-distended bladder is said to have happened during labour, in consequence of the attendant neglecting to relieve retention of urine ; more usually, the injury done to the bladder merely excites inflammation, which too often terminates in sloughing and the production of a fistula. The first accident must be a very hopeless one, the patient having scarcely a chance of escaping the low peritonitis that must be expected to ensue.

Ruptures of large blood-vessels in the abdomen, and lacerations of viscera, as the liver, &c., have been recorded. The symptoms will be obscure, and the nature of the case doubtful until after the death of the patient, and it is obvious that there will never be opportunity or encouragement for any medical treatment.

CHAPTER XIX.

MANAGEMENT OF PUERPERAL WOMEN.

IN ORDER to comprehend this subject, we must have clear ideas with respect to the state in which a woman is situated after labour. In the first place, her muscular power has been exerted in a violent and unusual manner probably for several hours, and as a natural consequence considerable fatigue produced ; secondly, her circulation has been a good deal excited, and a remarkable change has taken place in the relations of the abdominal viscera to each other and to their containing walls ; and, thirdly, the patient has been suffering more or less mental anxiety and distress.

All these circumstances manifestly require rest, both moral and physical ; and accordingly we must enjoin perfect quietude, and allow the woman to sleep, if she be inclined to do so. The erect posture, and every thing stimulating, either in the way of drink or food, must be positively forbidden, as, from the state of the circulation and of the abdomen, as well as of the nervous system, there is a peculiar liability to inflammatory or irritative action. Should the woman's stomach be empty, it will be well to give her some cold gruel or whey, with a little dry toast: this will employ her digestive organs, and prevent the very great annoyance which is sometimes experienced from flatulency. The binder will probably require a little tightening after the placenta has been expelled; the doubled sheet may then be drawn quietly from under the woman's hips, so as to make her more comfortable, and a dry folded napkin applied to the vulva. These precautions having been attended to, we may take our leave, giving strict directions that she shall not be moved at all for two or three hours, but that if she feel well at the end of that period, the left side of the bed may be arranged comfortably, and she may be shifted quietly upon it, so as to admit of the wet sheets, &c. being removed from the place where she was at first lying.

Within twelve hours we should always visit our patient, and we have then to ascertain the state of her tongue and pulse;* whether there be any pain or tenderness in the abdomen; whether she has

---

* The pulse should have fallen by this time from the elevation caused by the labour to nearly its natural standard. I have, however, found it to remain quick, in irritable women, for some days, without any bad results. These cases should be closely watched.

had sleep, and passed urine ; and whether the after pains have been severe, or the discharge copious. Should matters be going on well, we have nothing to do until twenty-four or thirty hours after delivery ; when, if the bowels have not been opened, a mild aperient of castor oil or rhubarb should be given, or an enema administered.*   A light, non-stimulant, but sufficiently nutritious, diet should be prescribed ; consisting, at first, of gruel, and tea or cocoa, with biscuits or toast.   On the third or fourth day, if nothing forbids, a little chicken may be allowed, and half a glass of white wine diluted with water; after which, a gradual, cautious return may be made to the ordinary diet.

The patient should not be allowed to rise from her bed sooner than the third or fourth day, and then only for a short time while it is being made. This restriction serves both to keep the circulation tranquil and to prevent prolapsus of the uterus, which is likely to happen, unless the parts are allowed time to regain their tone after the relaxation which they have suffered during parturition.   In

---

* When women have piles, castor oil often produces much irritation, and a preferable substitute will be a couple of drachms of senna electuary, or some of the infusion of senna with carbonate of magnesia, already mentioned. In ordinary cases, I would set my face entirely against the drastic purgatives sometimes employed. Nothing could be better devised for exciting intestinal irritation and fever than this unhappy practice.

the third week in summer, and probably the fourth in winter, a drive or walk in the open air may be permitted. All these limitations of time must of course be understood *cum grano salis,* and acted upon with reference to general principles. For instance, I have known it to be advisable to give solid food from the very first to patients with whose stomachs slops peculiarly disagreed. But of these matters, every practitioner must judge for himself; and in an acquaintance with such peculiarities and exceptions, derived from observation, consists that practical experience which teaches, but cannot be taught.

There are two secretions which play important parts in the woman's constitution after delivery— these are the lochia and the milk. The *lochia* consists at first merely of the blood which is squeezed out of the enlarged vessels by the contraction of the uterus. It continues sanguineous for some days, then changes to a greenish serum, finally becomes paler, and decreases gradually, until in three or four weeks (more or less, in different women) it altogether ceases. Like every other secretion, it is suppressed or diminished by any accession of fever or inflammation, and thus becomes a valuable diagnostic symptom of either of these states.

The existence of the lochia requires strict attention to cleanliness on the part of a puerperal woman and her attendants, as, if the discharge be allowed to accumulate, it soon becomes putrid and irritating. The vulva should be sponged every day with lukewarm water.

Milk commences to be secreted during the last days of gestation, and often much earlier. During the act of parturition, and for a few hours afterwards, a degree of fever exists, which often suspends the secretion for the time; but the popular notion, that it does not come until the third day, is quite unfounded, and leads to injurious practical results. After the woman has rested and slept a little (say in ten or twelve hours), the child may be applied to her breasts, generally with much advantage to herself and it. The constant removal of the milk as fast as it is secreted effectually prevents accumulation in the gland, and the distention and fever consequent upon it, which otherwise would happen about the third day, and the occurrence of which has given rise to the popular prejudice alluded to. If it be manifest, however, that there is no secretion in the breast, it is not advisable to keep the child applied, as its determined efforts to extract something may have the effect of excoriating the nipples, and creating much after-suffering.

The milk, like the lochia, is suppressed by fever or inflammation; and thus, by its quantity, it often affords useful indications. When a woman does not intend to nurse, her diet should consist less of fluids than under other circumstances; aperients should also be exhibited more freely; and if the breasts become hard and painful, they must be rubbed diligently with a little sweet oil, or perhaps it may be necessary to have the milk drawn from them by a breast pump.

After-pains.—These are rare after first labours, but they very commonly occur after subsequent ones: they are occasioned generally by the efforts of the uterus to expel coagula of blood, which from time to time collect in its cavity. They also seem to depend sometimes upon constipation. In some instances they continue from the time of delivery for several hours; in others, they do not commence until twelve, twenty-four, or thirty hours have elapsed.

We may distinguish these pains from peritoneal inflammation by their remissions, by the abdomen being free from remarkable tenderness, by the secretions of milk and lochia being undisturbed, and by the pulse being quiet and indicating no fever.

After-pains do not require much treatment; a little friction over the uterus, and a mild aperient, will often relieve them. When they are severe and prevent the woman from sleeping, it may be necessary to give an anodyne;* but, as the contractions

---

* Extracti Opii aquosi, gr. jss. in pilula; vel Tincturæ Opii, gtts. xxx. in haustu.

are a natural occurrence, and intended to remove coagula, which, if retained, might be injurious, it is as well, if we can so manage, to avoid a stoppage of the uterine action by narcotics.

Several accidents may happen during labour, which, after its completion, require to be understood and attended to by the accoucheur, although the treatment of many of them falls strictly within the province of surgery. Of these, we shall take a brief notice.

Lacerations of the perineum have been already alluded to : they may occur merely as rents of the posterior commissure of the vulva, or they may extend into the rectum ; or, lastly, the head of the child may be driven through the perineum, leaving the posterior commissure entire, and constituting what has been termed the circular perforation. In the first case, little treatment is required ; cleanliness should be strictly attended to, but there is no necessity for any dressing, as the sides of the wound are kept in apposition by the mere approximation of the thighs. When the injury is more severe, it becomes a case for surgical treatment, and therefore is beyond our present limits.

Inflammation of the vagina sometimes follows a tedious labour, or even a natural one, when the woman sits up too soon or too long at a time after delivery. The symptoms are heat and soreness of the part, with a sense of bearing down, and occasionally painful and frequent micturition. It may end in suppuration, and even adhesion of the vagina; or if the parts have, in the first instance, suffered much, there may result sloughing, and perhaps a fistulous communication with the bladder or rectum.

The inflammation must be treated in the commencement upon ordinary principles. The woman must be kept at rest, in the horizontal posture; fomentations should be applied, and the other means suitable to the case in a surgical point of view diligently employed. Our attentions should be redoubled if we see any reason to dread sloughing, which we may be led to expect when the woman is of a broken-down, bad constitution. In such a case, we should be particularly careful to draw off the urine, which should never be allowed to accumulate in the bladder.

Ecchymosis of the labia.—This sometimes occurs during a violent labour, in consequence of a bursting of some vessel, and consequent pouring out of blood into the loose cellular texture of which these parts are composed. A labium will sometimes become suddenly almost as large as the child's head, and may even impede delivery. In such a case it is recommended, immediately after the occurrence, to puncture the part, and allow the blood to escape while it is yet fluid.   This should never be done, however, after coagulation has taken place, as admission of the air then would cause the blood to become putrid, and excite a mischievous and unhealthy suppuration.   If we leave the part untouched, absorption will in time be effected, and no injurious consequence remain.

Retention of urine sometimes supervenes upon a perfectly natural labour in an irritable woman. In such cases, the urine must be drawn off twice a day with a catheter, until the bladder regains its tone, which it probably will in seven or eight days.   Should retention continue after the dangers of the puerperal state have been passed, it may be necessary to give tonics (especially preparations of iron), and to apply a blister to the sacrum.   These means are usually sufficient.

Incontinence of urine is also an occasional consequence of labour; but if there be no organic injury, it is not likely to be troublesome. The same *medical* treatment will apply to it as to retention.

Piles are sometimes productive of very great pain and inconvenience to puerperal women, the pressure upon them during labour causing inflammation and great tumefaction.   Warm fomentations will often give sufficient relief, but occasionally it is necessary to apply leeches.   Eight or ten may be put on, and when they fall off, may be succeeded by a warm poultice of chamomile flowers, which will encourage the bleeding, and give much relief. I have already alluded to the kind of aperients best suited for piles, and mentioned that castor oil, contrary to what is commonly supposed, is very likely to irritate the extremity of the rectum.*

Obstacles to nursing.—One of the most formidable of these arises from a deficiency of nipple. Owing to the tight dresses worn by women, this part is sometimes so firmly compressed into the substance of the breast, as to offer nothing for the child's lips to lay hold of. In such a case it must be drawn out by the breast pump, or by the lips of a strong child, and the infant instantly applied.

Sore nipples.—The nipples of some women are peculiarly tender, and liable to excoriation. When we know that this is the case before labour, we should harden them by exposure to the air for some time every morning, and by the use of a lotion of spirits and water. The only effectual means of relief, when excoriations do occur, is the use of the nipple shield, whereby the exciting cause (pressure of the child's mouth) is removed.† In

---

* When the inflammation has subsided, I have seen much benefit derived from the following liniment, recommended by Mr. Colles: a drachm of laudanum may be added to it with advantage. ℞ Olei Olivarum, ℥ij.; Liquoris Subacet. Plumbi, ℥j. M. Fiat linimentum.

† The best form of this useful instrument is that made of gum elastic.

addition to this, we may apply slightly stimulating lotions, as sulphate of zinc solution,* or spirits and water, or, what answers very well, the black wash; care being taken to cleanse the nipples from any of these substances before the child is again allowed to touch them. Syphilitic sores, or aphthæ, may be communicated from the child's mouth to the nipples, and, of course, from their specific nature, they demand peculiar attention.

* ℞ Sulphatis Zinci, gr. viij.; Aquæ Rosarum, ℥iv. M. Fiat lotio.

The following, I believe, is a formula of Sir A. Cooper's, and is very useful :—℞ Subborat. Sodæ, ℨij.; Cretæ precipitatæ, ℥j.; Sp. Rectificati, Aquæ Rosarum, āā ℥iij. M. Fiat lotio.

CHAPTER XX.

PUERPERAL FEVER.

UNDER THIS NAME authors have described several
modifications of disease, and even some totally
distinct affections, thereby causing so much confusion, that many gentlemen have been induced to
contrive, in its stead, a variety of terms, by which
they hoped not only to designate a certain malady,
but to convey scientific allusions as to its nature.
In the complete attainment of these objects, I think
they have all failed, and I shall therefore continue
to employ the old term*, as involving no peculiar
theory, and as being now perfectly well understood

---

* It has always appeared to me, that the more hieroglyphical
we can make our terms, the better, in so uncertain a science as
medicine. When a name contains a theory, it must lead us
astray as soon as the latter is changed; and how long does any
theory hold its ground in pathology? If authors sought to
obtain and teach correct *ideas* of the *nature* of diseases under
their old names, in place of inventing new ones, we should have
less of that fighting about words, which is unquestionably the
opprobrium of medicine.

to apply to a certain range of very fatal morbid conditions which occasionally follow parturition.

Diseases properly termed Puerperal Fevers, and coming strictly within the meaning which we wish to apply to these words, may occur either sporadically, or as very destructive and general epidemics; and under these different forms they have been repeatedly described with variously modified symptoms, and as often treated by excellent practitioners upon diametrically opposite principles. So various, indeed, have been the accounts of writers, that no symptoms can be fixed upon as having been commonly described by all, excepting fever, quick pulse, and tenderness (often very indistinct) in the abdomen. Amid these bewildering circumstances we must seek our guide, both for theory and practice, in an attentive consideration of the pathology of the disease, upon which subject the profession is much indebted to the researches of Dr. S. Cusack and Dr. Lee. By both these gentlemen, the affection is considered as an inflammation occurring within the abdomen; and by the latter, it is supposed, that the various forms which it assumes, ' whether inflammatory, congestive, or typhoid, in a great measure depend on whether the serous, muscular, or venous tissue of the organ has become affected.' This proposition is probably, to a certain extent, correct; but as Dr. Lee's divisions are rather suited to the dissecting room than the sick chamber, we shall take Dr. Cusack's more practical classification into three species:—1. the Inflammatory; 2. the Typhoid; and 3. the Mixed.

1. The first or inflammatory species differs but little from ordinary peritonitis. It occurs in patients of good constitution, and, when epidemic, prevails simultaneously with diseases of a decidedly sthenic character. Its causes are exposure to cold, irregularities in diet, and perhaps contagion.

The symptoms are, first, a rigor, seizing the patient usually about the second, third, or fourth day after labour; if the abdomen be carefully examined, some tenderness will immediately be found over the uterus, which quickly increases to severe pain, and extends over the whole abdomen. The pain may be aggravated in paroxysms, but is never absent, and the tenderness becomes in a short time so exquisite, that the patient cannot bear even the weight of the bed-clothes. She lies upon her back with her knees drawn up, so as to relax, as much as possible, the abdominal walls; and, in order to avoid the pressure of the diaphragm, endeavours to respire by means of the intercostal muscles, thus giving to the breathing a very laboured character. The rigors are succeeded by nausea, heat of skin, thirst, and often intense pain in the forehead. The countenance is expressive of great suffering. The pulse is quick, sometimes full and throbbing, at others hard and wiry, but always *incompressible.* The tongue is generally white and creamy, but varies in its appearance. The bowels are usually constipated, the urine scanty, and the milk and lochia suppressed. If the disease be allowed to run on, the belly becomes tympanitic, diarrhœa and vomiting of dark matter ensue, the pulse becomes feeble, the breathing hurried, sometimes with severe pain in the chest, and death occurs about the fourth day, often much sooner.

The disease is liable to be confounded with severe after-pains, intestinal irritation, and hysteric tenderness of the uterus and abdomen. From the first, it is to be distinguished by its want of remissions, by the tenderness on pressure, and by the severity of the fever. Intestinal irritation is to be known chiefly by the previous marks of derangement of the chylopoietic viscera, and by the absence of extreme tenderness, on pressure. In hysteric tenderness, it is often very difficult to discriminate, the patient appearing to suffer exquisite torture, and screaming even before our hand reaches the surface of her body. In these cases, however, if we are able to divert away the woman's attention, and, still keeping our hand upon the abdomen, to gradually increase the pressure, we shall find that she can easily bear what she at first shrank from with terror.

The morbid appearances in this species are precisely similar to those observable in peritonitis. The peritoneum, especially near the uterus, is thickened, vascular, and coated with lymph; the viscera are frequently agglutinated together, and there is an effusion into the cavity (often in immense quantity) of whey-coloured or sero-purulent fluid, mixed with flakes or masses of lymph. The omentum is sometimes inflamed, and there is a large quantity of air both in the intestines and abdominal cavity. In the thoracic cavity there may be serous effusion into the bronchial cellular tissue and pleura, or a coating of lymph upon the latter.

2. The typhoid form of the disease occurs in patients of broken-down constitutions and depressed minds, living in unhealthy situations, and who probably have suffered from hemorrhage or manual interference with the interior of the uterus. When epidemic, it appears to prevail in connection with diseases of an asthenic character, as typhus fever, erysipelas, and diffuse inflammation; and, like these, it often occasions sad ravages in hospitals.

The symptoms are by no means so prominent as in the first species: there is often little or no pain, and scarcely any tenderness, except at the commencement, and then perhaps only when we press firmly upon the uterus. The disease usually commences with a rigor, but even this is sometimes indistinct. The pulse is quick and feeble, and differs from its character in the first species by being remarkably *compressible*. There is extreme weakness and exhaustion, with want of rest; of all which the countenance is particularly expressive. Indeed, so remarkable is the anxiety apparent in the patient's face from the very outset, that one can often recognise the disease from the appearance of it alone. The skin is also sallow and dirty-looking, and seldom hot; towards the close there may be petechiæ. The respiration is hurried —the lochia and milk suppressed, or the former diminished and fœtid. In the latter stages there is often a feculent diarrhœa. The tongue is sometimes natural, and remarkably clean, or it may be of a bluish creamy whiteness, or even blackish.

The patient quickly becomes weaker and weaker, and the disease may proceed to a fatal termination in a few hours, or it may hang on for twelve or fourteen days. In some instances I have had a firm conviction that this form of fever had made its commencement several days before parturition, and that in many cases where it was supposed to be the consequence, it was, in fact, the cause of difficult labour.

The morbid appearances in this species differ considerably from those observed in the first, but still they are obviously the result of a kind of inflammation. The effusion into the peritoneal cavity is by no means so great as in the former affection, nor are there any adhesions or extravasations of lymph. The fluid effused is sometimes a brownish, dirty-looking serum ; at others, of an oily, semi-purulent character. In the subserous and pelvic cellular tissue, and between the broad ligaments, a reddish serum or a gelatinous fluid is deposited in considerable quantity. The same deposits often exist in the uterine substance, which may be softened and altered in texture, so as to present a gangrenous appearance, and may contain depositions of pus. The internal coat of the womb is also sometimes softened in patches, and of a dark or ash-grey colour. Similar changes may occasionally be observed in the coats of the intestines. The ovaries are frequently enlarged and changed into cysts of pus, and may undergo a process of softening to such a degree as not to admit of being handled without being destroyed. The absorbents and veins of the uterus, in some cases, are found filled wth pus ; and abscesses and disorganisation may occur simultaneously in distant organs, as the lungs, spleen, liver, joints, eyes, brain, &c. ; the disease in these melancholy examples strikingly resembling that form of diffuse inflammation which follows dissection wounds, or operations performed upon unhealthy subjects during the prevalence of erysipelas. Dr. Lee has divided the morbid appearances just described into three sections, considering that the disease may distinctly affect the appendages of the uterus, its muscular tissue, or its veins and absorbents. He has not, however, been able to point out any means of diagnosis between these, nor any difference in the effects of remedies, or in the ordinary fatal results. His division, in fact, is founded upon morbid anatomy, not upon pathology, and therefore is not of use in practice.

3. There is decidedly a mixed species of the disease; what, in fact, we might expect to meet with in an individual of strong constitution, at a time when the 'constitutio anni' was of an asthenic type.

The symptoms are a mixture of those of the other two : considerable pain and tenderness often existing, with a pulse not possessing the wiry hardness or incompressibility of the inflammatory species; much debility and little relief following the employment of the lancet; and the blood neither presenting the highly inflammatory appearance of the first form, nor the broken-down, scarcely coagulating quality of the second.

The morbid appearances generally indicate inflammation of the peritoneum, but wanting the very adhesive character of the first species, and often presenting at the same time a degree of the sub-serous infiltration and tendency to alteration in the uterine appendages which characterise the typhoid form.

Some difference of opinion has existed as to the contagious or non-contagious nature of puerperal fever. Like every question of the kind, it is one extremely difficult to come to any conclusion about. But so many instances have been recorded of the disease following a particular nurse or accoucheur, that it would be now highly culpable in any practitioner not to adopt the most strict precautions against the risk of his carrying infection from one patient to another. After seeing a case of this fever, the clothes should always be changed, the most careful ablutions performed, and no accoucheur should personally interfere in the opening of the bodies of victims to the complaint. Should a run of fever continue to affect the patients of any individual, notwithstanding attention to these matters, it becomes his bounden duty to abstain temporarily from practice, and, if possible, to remove for a time from his ordinary residence.

The *treatment* of puerperal fever, of course, varies very much according to the species.

In the inflammatory form, antiphlogistic treatment is decidedly indicated in the commencement, and the lancet should be our sheet-anchor. As much blood (probably from twelve to twenty-four ounces) must be taken from the arm as will produce a decided effect upon the circulation. To do this most efficiently, a large orifice should be made in a vein, while the patient is in a recumbent posture, its effects upon the pulse and countenance being carefully watched. Dr. Cusack very justly remarks, that placing the woman in the erect posture when we are going to bleed her, will generally produce syncope, quite independently of the abstraction of blood, and may prevent the useful employment of this remedy. We must be guided, with respect to a repetition of venesection, by the effect of the first, and by the appearance of the blood. The latter, and the compressibility or non-compressibility of the pulse, afford very valuable indications. When there is any doubt about a second blood-letting, we may, as an intermediate measure, apply leeches to the abdomen. Venesection, when it is proper, should always be adopted as early as possible in the complaint, as the lapse of a very brief space of time may render its employment worse than useless. As long, however, as the pulse retained its *incompressibility*, I should not be prevented from using the lancet, even by the existence of considerable debility; the former symptom, I think, giving the truest indication upon this point.

After bleeding, whether we think it advisable to apply leeches or not, we shall find great advantage from a fomentation of the whole abdomen with spirits of turpentine,* or the application of a

---

* To apply this, a piece of flannel may be wrung out of hot water, and an ounce or two of the turpentine sprinkled upon it.

bag of scalded bran or chamomile flowers, as hot as can be borne. Either of these latter are infinitely preferable to poultices, from their lightness and cleanliness. The turpentine has often a peculiarly good effect, removing distressing flatulency, and sometimes producing evacuations from the bowels. If constipation exists, a smart purgative, as castor oil and spirits of turpentine (half an ounce of each), or a bolus of jalap and calomel (ten grains of the former, and five of the latter), may be administered, and followed by an enema. Should the bolus be given, and not act quickly, it must be assisted by a purgative mixture (inf. sennæ, &c.). If the stomach be irritable, it may be more advisable to give the purgative in the form of pills.* When the constipation has been relieved, the intestinal canal should not be further irritated by cathartics. After bleeding, and freeing the bowels, the next remedies upon which our dependence should be placed are decidedly calomel and opium. The former should be given in doses of two or three grains every second hour, until the system is influenced, combining one-sixth or one-fourth of a grain of opium, should the

It causes great pain, of which the patient should be apprised, and warned to remove it as soon as the smarting becomes very severe.

　* ℞ Extract. Colocynth. comp. ℈ss.; Calomelanos, gr. x.; Olei Caryophill. gs. iii. Ft. massa, et divide in pilulas decem: sumantur duæ 2ᵈᵃ q.q. horâ ad effectum.

bowels be irritable. At night, ten grains of Dover's powder will often be found to produce sleep, and do much service. When the mouth becomes affected, the prognosis is almost always favourable, and we should continue the action by giving smaller doses of mercury.

I have no great opinion of the use of blisters in abdominal inflammations, especially in the first stages, as they then very effectually deprive us of one of our best guides, by masking the pain and tenderness upon pressure. In the latter stages, however, they are often of service.

The regimen, in this species, must, of course, be rigidly antiphlogistic : and, should the disease subside, the strictest precautions must be adopted to prevent relapse, to which there is a considerable tendency.

In the second species, bleeding is always injurious, and often hastens a fatal termination.

The medicines upon which most reliance can be placed in this very intractable malady are mercury and opium; and, as a very great source of suffering exists in the patient's restlessness and want of sleep, the latter drug may be given in considerable doses; for example, a grain every three or four hours, in combination with from two to four grains of calomel, until the patient sleeps, or an effect is produced upon the system by the mercury. According to the observations of Drs. Graves and

Stokes,* opium appears to exercise a beneficial
influence in several low forms of inflammation,
and there is a good deal of encouragement for its
free use in this disease.   If the bowels are constipated, or we have reason to suppose them to be
loaded, a mild aperient must be given; but it
should be of a warm and simply laxative kind, as
the rhubarb draught already mentioned.† Spirit
of turpentine has been recommended by some
gentlemen, and it will sometimes be found of use
by acting as an aperient, and, at the same time,
stimulating and restoring a healthy tone to the
mucous membrane.‡ We should be extremely
cautious about giving any drastic purgative, lest
it might increase the debility and accelerate the
approach of diarrhœa, which is often a very
troublesome symptom.   When the latter sets in,
we must endeavour to check it by enemata of
starch and laudanum.   The application of turpentine, externally, will often be of service; and
we may, also, in the progress of the complaint,
employ blisters with more advantage' than in the
inflammatory species.

The dietetic and general management of the

* Vide Dublin Hosp. Reports, vol. v.
† Vide p. 101.
‡ ℞ Sp. Terebinthinæ rect. ℥vj.; Aquæ Cinnamomi, ℥vj.;
Syrupi Zingiberis, ℥j. M. Fiat haustus 2ᵈᵃ quâque horâ
sumend.

patient is of much importance. She should, if possible, be placed in an open airy room; wine must be given, diluted with water, or in arrow-root, so as cautiously to support the strength, taking care, at the same time, not to add to the gastric derangement. Cold chicken broth may be allowed as ordinary drink, and will be often found to agree remarkably well with the stomach.

Should a rally be made, we shall be obliged to assist the patient's recovery by light tonics, and, perhaps, by sulphate of quinine. At all times we must be carefully on the watch for a relapse.

The third or mixed species of puerperal fever requires a modified and cautious treatment. Our principal reliance must be upon calomel and opium; but, although general blood-letting is seldom safe, we shall frequently find much advantage in the application of leeches (two or three dozen) to the hypogastrium, repeating them, according to the degree of pain and tenderness, and the manner in which the loss of blood is borne.

In the treatment of all these species, we are to recollect that the one frequently runs into the other, and that they must always be managed according to the symptoms, and not upon any preconceived notion respecting their type. To no malady, indeed, is the excellent advice of Sydenham more appropriate, 'to find out, in the first place, the genius of epidemic diseases, which, though they may seem alike to the unwary, because in some sort they do agree, to outward appearance, yet, if seriously considered, are very different.'

Emetics, antimonial preparations, and various other remedies of all kinds, have, as might have been expected in so fatal a disease, been recommended for the treatment of puerperal fever; but, my object being simply to give a plain statement of what I conceive to be useful in practice, I think it would be exceeding my limits to enter into the consideration of speculations of this kind, which are not supported by solid practical foundations.

CHAPTER XXI.

ORDINARY FEVERS OF PUERPERAL WOMEN.

THE IRRITABILITY of the nervous system and of certain organs, always more or less attendant upon the puerperal condition, render women liable to a number of febrile affections, besides the formidable disease treated of in the last chapter.

One of the most common of these is the *ephemera*, or *weed*. This fever sets in generally during the first three or four days after parturition, with a severe rigor. It consists of a cold, hot, and sweating stage, and may terminate in twenty-four hours, having but one paroxysm. The rigor is often very severe and long continued. During the hot stage there is intense headache, intolerance of light, quick, but otherwise good pulse, great thirst, white and coated tongue. Sometimes there is slight abdominal tenderness, and the bowels are generally confined. The sweating in the third stage is profuse, and the symptoms continue very much as in the second. After some hours, the symptoms begin to subside, the patient probably falls asleep, and awakes convalescent. In other cases, the duration of the fever is not so short: other paroxysms (though not so violent as the first) succeed, and the disease may hang on for eight or ten days, constituting what may be called *Intestinal fever*. Weed may be distinguished from puerperal fever by a want of the tenderness so remarkable in the inflammatory form of that disease, by the regularity of its stages, its history, and by the general contrast that will be observed upon a careful examination of all the symptoms.

The causes of the ephemera, or intestinal fever, are to be found in an irritated state of the intestinal mucous membrane and derangement of the hepatic system, usually occasioned by irregularities of diet, exposure to cold, &c. Among the lower classes of people nothing is more common than to find weed excited by drinking porter or spirits shortly after delivery; and corresponding irregularities among the rich are attended by similar results.

From what has been said of the causes, the treatment must be obvious. Should it have arisen from the taking of improper food, and our attention be directed to this circumstance at an early period, we may hope to cut short the complaint by the ad-

ministration of a mild emetic of ipecacuan. Afterwards, or, without using the emetic, should we not
have seen the patient in the commencement, we
must set the bowels and hepatic system right by
the administration of a purgative, containing some
mercurial: three grains of calomel, or five grains
of hydrargyrus cum cretâ, with perhaps a little
antimonial powder, may be given, and followed
by a senna mixture or a rhubarb draught, according
to the circumstances of the case.   When we see a
patient during the rigor, we must endeavour to
restore warmth, and bring on the hot stage by
giving warm diluents, and applying heat to the
feet.   In the sweating stage, we must ventilate
the room and lighten the bed-clothes, without,
however, exposing the woman to any risk of cold.
If the headache be severe, or anything more than
a very slight abdominal tenderness exist, it will be
erring on the safe side to apply leeches respectively
either to the head or belly.   Should the fever not
terminate at once, our further attentions must be
directed to the re-establishment of a healthy tone
in the bowels, by careful watching of the secretions,
and by the enforcement of a mild, unirritating
regimen.   In the progress of intestinal fever, the
bowels may become loose, and the abdomen somewhat tender and tumid; the case, in fact, very
much resembling the remittent fever of children.

Change of air, and the continued use of mild alterative mercurials (as the hyd. cum cretâ *) with light bitters (as the infusion of colombo), when the tongue begins to clean, will be the remedies most likely to serve.

.It is remarkable that the milk and lochia may continue to be secreted during the existence of this fever. It is almost needless to say, that the most careful attention must be paid to any symptoms of local mischief that may show themselves, either in the abdomen or head.

Miliary fever.—When the ephemera, or intestinal fever, has been mismanaged, the patient being kept in a heated, ill-ventilated apartment, and the bowels not set to rights, a miliary eruption occasionally supervenes.

This eruption consists of a number of small papulæ, resembling millet seeds, upon the apex of which little vesicles form, containing a fluid at first straw-coloured, and subsequently becoming white or yellow. In two or three days these scab and desquamate, and other crops probably succeed. The papulæ first appear upon the forehead, neck, and breast—rarely upon the face. Two varieties, a red and white, are described, of which the former is said to be the mildest. Before the eruption the skin becomes rough, and there is a sen-

---

* ℞ Pil. Rhei comp. ℨss.; Hyd. cum Cretâ ℈j. Fiat massa, et divide in pilulas x.: sum. ij. 2ᵈᵃ quâque nocte.

sation in it of prickling heat: after it has appeared there are frequently other marks of derangement of the mucous membrane, as aphthæ in the mouth, and red-edged tongue. The patient is generally bathed in a profuse acid perspiration.

The treatment is that recommended in intestinal fever, but, as there is usually more debility, bark and mineral acids will probably be required in the latter stages. For further information upon miliary fever, which is not a peculiarly puerperal disease, reference must be made to systematic works upon the practice of physic.

Milk fever.—When the milk begins to be secreted copiously, there is always some degree of febrile excitement. Should the milk be allowed to accumulate, in consequence of the woman declining to nurse, or the child being improperly withheld, this excitement becomes an actual fever, ushered in by rigors, and followed by hot and sweating stages, with all the *et cetera* described under the head of ephemera. In addition, there is a distended and very painful state of the breasts.

A smart purgative will be required to allay the fever, but the natural and obvious remedy is, of course, to remove the offending secretion. For this purpose the child should be applied early, or, if that be not practicable, the breast must be diligently and gently rubbed with a soft hand, and a little sweet oil, until the milk runs from it; or the breast pump may be employed to draw it. Where the woman does not intend to nurse, it is better to avoid the latter, as it tends to excite a continuance of the secretion.

The danger in this fever is, that it may terminate in mammary abscess, a most painful and distressing complaint. When we have reason to dread its supervention, from the severity of the fever, the most effectual treatment is to nauseate the patient with tartar emetic. A grain or two of this medicine may be given in the purgative mixture which we usually have occasion to exhibit at the commencement, and if that does not succeed, it may be subsequently given in solution, in doses of an eighth or sixteenth of a grain, every half hour, until nausea is produced. When a patient is not about to nurse, purgatives must be occasionally used, until the secretion altogether ceases, and she must be cautioned to remain quiet, and to avoid putting on stays, or any other tight dress, that may press upon the mammæ, while they are in an excited condition. If a mammary abscess be unavoidable, we must promote suppuration by fomentations, &c.* according to the plans laid down by surgical writers.

---

* The best mode of fomenting the breast is by placing upon it a piece of flannel wrung out of hot water, and over that a wooden bowl (somewhat larger than the gland) which has been heated in boiling water; by this plan a sort of steam bath is formed, and all injurious pressure avoided.

CHAPTER XXII.

PHLEGMASIA DOLENS.

THIS painful affection generally attacks women between the tenth and sixteenth days after delivery, seldom earlier, but sometimes at a much later period. Its subjects are generally persons of broken-down constitutions, and it frequently attacks those who have suffered from hemorrhage or manual interference with the interior of the uterus, and in whom, before its invasion, there are manifest signs of irritation of that organ.

The disease is usually ushered in by distinct febrile symptoms: there is a rigor, followed by heat, thirst, loaded tongue, full pulse, and headache. The cause of these symptoms is soon revealed, by the occurrence of pain and stiffness in one of the groins, upper part of the thigh, or labium; or the pain may first be felt in the knee or calf of the leg. This is rapidly succeeded by tumefaction, which spreads from the point first attacked, and, within twenty-four or forty-eight hours, the limb is sometimes increased to nearly

twice its original size. There is then exquisite
pain, aggravated by the slightest attempt at motion.
The limb is tense, white, and shining, is elastic to
the touch, and pits very little upon pressure, but
gives to the hand passed over it a sense of irregularity, as if it contained numerous little depres-
sions under the tense integument. The swelling,
in some instances, goes on slowly, not arriving at
its maximum for several days. When the whole
extremity is swelled, the violence of the pain abates,
but it is still very severe upon the least effort at
motion, and the patient loses all command over
the limb. The temperature is increased, and there
is a good deal of pain upon pressure, which is
said to be greater along the course of the veins,
but I cannot say that I have observed this to be
always the case. At this time, there is a good
deal of fever, with a quick, feeble pulse, white
tongue, and pale face. The lochia are suppressed,
or diminished and fetid, and the urine is muddy.
The patient suffers greatly from want of sleep. In
six or eight days (more or less in different cases),
the febrile symptoms begin to abate, and the
swelling slowly diminishes; first in the thigh, and
afterwards in the leg and foot. As tumefaction
decreases, the veins, absorbents, and lymphatic
glands may sometimes be discovered enlarged and
indurated, and the limb begins to pit upon pressure, more than it previously did. The patient

remains weak and feeble, with very little power over her leg, which feels heavy, stiff, and benumbed. The disease is generally, at first, confined to one extremity and labium, but it frequently extends to the other. The ultimate recovery is very slow, and there may be a fatal termination, the patient being worn down by the protracted constitutional disturbance, or by extensive suppurations and purulent depôts, which occasionally form in the affected limb.

The pathology of phlegmasia dolens is still extremely obscure. By the older writers it was supposed to be an irregular deposit of the milk (*dépôt du lait*); by others, an extravasation of lymph, in consequence of rupture of the lymphatics; and, by some, a general inflammatory state of the same class of vessels. None of these hypotheses account for the symptoms, nor are they supported by *post-mortem* observations. I cannot avoid expressing the same opinion with respect to Dr. Davis's idea, that the disease is phlebitis of the crural veins. Phlegmasia dolens is well known not to be in general a fatal disease, and it is equally notorious that phlebitis in any part of the body is especially mortal. Besides this objection, I cannot see that the phenomena of the disease are satisfactorily explainable upon the idea of its being venous inflammation. In the generality of cases of the latter malady, there is nothing corresponding to the peculiar firm swelling of phlegmasia dolens, and an attentive examination of Dr. Lee's cases of actual phlebitis will show that they were very distinguishable from the other disease. I do not mean to deny, however, that inflammation and suppuration of the veins is often to be found upon examination of the bodies of those who have died of phlegmasia dolens, but it appears to me that the evidence already in existence does not prove that this inflammation is the cause of the swelled leg, but merely that it supervenes, in certain cases, upon that disease. The disease appears to me to consist in an inflammation of the cellular tissue, occasioning an effusion of coagulating lymph ; but how the inflammation is excited, or why it produces those peculiar effects, has not yet been discovered.

The prognosis, when the disease is uncomplicated, is favourable, but recovery is always slow and very protracted.

The treatment in the acute state must be conducted upon the antiphlogistic plan. The nature of the fever and circumstances of the patient, however, generally forbid the use of the lancet, and we usually find it advisable to trust to the application of leeches to the groin and to those parts where the pain is chiefly seated. One or two dozen may be applied at first, and subsequently a smaller number repeated, if necessary, pursuing the pain, as it were, into the different localities in which it may lurk. The bleeding may be encouraged by warm fomentation with decoction of poppy heads or infusion of chamomile, which latter measure of itself does great service. In some rare cases, more benefit will be derived from the use of evaporating lotions. As the bowels are frequently constipated, we shall probably have occasion to employ an aperient, but it should be of a mild warm kind;* and it is not necessary that its effects should be very powerful. As the patient's nights are generally sleepless, we shall find great advantage from giving ten grains of Dover's powder and two or three of calomel at bed-time. I think it is generally advisable to give calomel and antimonial powder, so as slightly to affect the mouth, but I should by no means recommend any attempt at speedy salivation. A grain of each three times a day, with the addition of two or three grains of Dover's powder, should the bowels not be confined, will be quite sufficient. The regimen should be antiphlogistic, and strict rest enjoined. After the inflammation has subsided, we must alter our hand, and endeavour judiciously to improve the tone of the constitution. A light nutritious diet may be allowed, change of air, or at all events free ventilation obtained, and the digestive organs improved

* As the infusion of senna, or the rhubarb draught, already specified.

by the use of light bitters and mineral acids.* While we are acting in this way, however, we shall frequently have to attend to recurring signs of local inflammation, and should always meet them by the application of leeches. The limb must be still kept at perfect rest, in a horizontal position ; but when it is able to bear slight frictions with the hand, these will be found serviceable, as will also sponging with tepid salt water : at a later period bandaging and strapping the limb with adhesive plaster may be used. We shall often have occasion for all our in- genuity in contriving plans of treatment, as the feeble state of the part may continue for months or even years. When depositions of pus are ascertained to exist in any part of the extremity, free incisions are required to give exit to the matter, the more particularly as it is generally diffused through the cellular and other tissues, and seldom confined by a regular cyst. These cases of abscess are at- tended usually with very low typhoid fever, and frequently require the exhibition of wine, opium, camphor, quinine, and ammonia.

---

* ℞ Inf. Cascarillæ, Mist. Camphoræ, aa. ʒiij.; Sodæ Sub- carb. ʒss.; Sp. Ammon. aromat. gs. xxx. M. Sum. ʒj. ter quotidie.

CHAPTER XXIII.

PUERPERAL MANIA.

THIS OCCURS in two forms, the maniacal and melancholic, and makes its appearance, generally, within the first few days after labour. A similar disease may also happen when the woman has been exhausted by a continuance of the process of nursing longer than is suitable to her strength. The disease is most likely to attack persons of a nervous susceptible temperament, and whose minds have been shaken by depressing passions, or other causes of mental emotion. 'A large proportion of cases,' Dr. Gooch states, 'have occurred in patients in whose families disordered mind had already appeared.'

With respect to the cause, nothing more explicit can be stated than the opinion of the same distinguished writer, that it exists in the peculiar nervous excitement which, more or less, accompanies all the actions of the generative system.

The attack is sometimes quite sudden, but more generally the patient may be observed for some time previously to be irritable and peevish, or melancholy and gloomy, with a pulse somewhat quickened, and evident marks of disorder of the digestive organs, as furred tongue, yellow conjunctiva, and costive bowels. The derangement of mind is very various; in one case the patient being gloomy and desponding, while in another she is so violent as to require the employment of coercion, talking and moving about incessantly, and scarcely ever sleeping. In many instances, there is a very strong disposition to commit suicide. The bodily symptoms are those already mentioned, denoting derangement of the chylopoietic viscera. The pulse is quickened, but not usually to any remarkable degree; and it has been remarked by Dr. Gooch, that a very rapid pulse is a particularly unfavourable sign. The face is most commonly pale, and there does not exist, in ordinary cases, any evidence of inflammation or congestion of the brain.

The prognosis is generally favourable, but in some cases, especially those in which there is a quick weak pulse, with extreme watchfulness, a state of exhaustion may be produced that will ultimately prove fatal. The probability of complete mental recovery is also considerable, and there are not many chances in favour of a return of the disease in future labours.

The treatment of puerperal mania must be both

medical and moral. The former requires very nice discrimination, in order to adapt our measures to the exigencies of each particular case. General blood-letting is very seldom admissible, and never required, unless there exist manifest tokens of congestion or inflammation of the parts within the cranium. Even where these ·exist to a certain extent, it will be better, if possible, to meet them by local than by constitutional depletion, and the utmost ordinarily required is the application of a few leeches to the temples. In such cases nauseating doses of tartar emetic may often be employed with advantage. Attention to the intestinal canal will always be requisite, but the kind and degree of it must depend upon the peculiar circumstances of the case. If there be a loaded tongue, a yellow eye, and offensive breath, all indicating the stomach as the seat of irritation, a mild emetic of ipecacuan will often be of signal service. This may be followed by a purgative, or, where the former is not admissible, the latter may be administered at once, and should be of such a nature as will produce evacuations without exciting much secretion from the mucous membrane.*

* Dr. Gooch recommends for this purpose the aloetic pill, or compound decoction of aloes. I must here acknowledge that gentleman's excellent paper as the source from which the above brief sketch of puerperal mania was chiefly drawn. To that essay, as indeed to the whole of his writings, the reader's attention may be directed, upon his own principle, as to the work of

From the want of sleep suffered by the patient, it is obvious that narcotics are indicated, and accordingly we shall find our most valuable remedies in that class of medicines. It will be, of course, advisable to see that there is no great vascular excitement before we use them, and it will generally be necessary to premise laxatives. The black drop will be found to be one of the best forms in which we can administer opium. A full dose (say twelve drops) may be given, and repeated in an hour or two if it fail to produce sleep. Smaller doses may be subsequently employed, to keep up the calm produced by the first. Should the stomach bear it, the Dover's powder will also be found very serviceable ; and if it be necessary to vary the medicine, extract of hyoscyamus and camphor may be given together, in a dose of five grains of each. In the latter stages of the complaint, when the vascular excitement has entirely subsided, it will be necessary to have recourse to light bitters and mineral acids, for the purpose of improving the patient's general health.

The diet ought always to be sufficiently nutritious; of course, it must be of a light and unheating kind, and given with due regard to the disordered state of the digestive organs. In some

‘ a master mind, which we return to again and again, not merely for the knowledge which it contains, but to observe how that mind worked.’

instances wine may be beneficial ; its use, of course, is to be regulated according to the judgment of the practitioner. When the disease occurs in individuals weakened by protracted nursing, there is a still more imperative demand upon our discretion, in the avoidance of everything that may unnecessarily lower the strength.

The moral management should be intrusted to persons accustomed to the care of the insane. In the first instance, the patient should be put under the charge of a nurse of this description, by whom she should be closely watched, and every instrument that might be employed for the purpose of suicide must be carefully put out of reach. When the disease is likely to be protracted, it becomes a question as to whether it may be advisable to place the woman entirely in the hands of a physician who makes it his business to treat insanity. On this point, of course, no general rules can be laid down ; the taking of such a step, and the mode of taking it, must altogether depend upon the circumstances of the case. Dr. Gooch forbids all intercourse with the husband ; but I lately heard of a case in which this rule was not adhered to, and yet rather good effects attended its violation.

Actual phrenitis occasionally occurs during the puerperal state, and requires a treatment of course essentially different from that just laid down. Instead of the supporting and tranquillising system generally adapted to puerperal mania, the most active depletion will be required in phrenitis, and will too often fail of success. The treatment of this formidable disease does not come within my purpose, and it is only mentioned, to remind the reader of the necessity of discriminating justly between it and puerperal mania.

NOTE

ON THE MEANS OF RESUSCITATING STILL-BORN CHILDREN.

IN ADDITION to the measures recommended for this purpose at p. 107, viz. tickling the mouth and fauces, rubbing and gently slapping the chest, and allowing the funis to bleed, we are advised by most obstetric authors to employ the warm bath and artificial inflation of the lungs. Recent enquiries, however, have thrown considerable doubt upon the propriety of adopting either of these measures. According to Dr. Edwards's experiments, the warm bath must act injuriously, by excluding the atmospheric air, which he found to play a most important part in the removal of asphyxia. Again, the observations of MM. Leroy and Majendie prove 'that brisk inflation of air into the trachea killed rabbits, foxes, goats, sheep, and other animals, even when the force employed was that of an expiration from the human lungs,' and that 'from the records kept in the city of

Paris of the results of means employed for the recovery of persons drowned, the greater prevalence of the practice of insufflation has been coincident with a decrease of the number restored to life.' * Mr. Porter, who performed experiments similar to those of Leroy, and with like results, before he knew of the investigations of that gentleman, mentioned to me the fact that insufflation of cold air from a bellows, in the event of the person's resuscitation, seldom fails to produce dangerous bronchitis. From a consideration of these circumstances, I would recommend heat to be applied to a still-born infant, by holding it before a fire upon a person's lap; the chest and abdomen to be well rubbed with warm, dry flannel; and the nostrils and fauces to be tickled with a feather dipped in spirits. The lungs may be filled once or twice, by the operator applying his lips, with a bit of silk or muslin intervening (for the sake of cleanliness) to those of the child, and gently breathing into its mouth. While doing this, the nostrils must be held between the finger and thumb of one hand, and the fingers of the other should be placed upon the pit of the stomach, so as to prevent the air from passing into that organ. When the chest has been distended, it may be compressed gently with the hand, so as again to

* Review of Dr. Kay's work on Asphyxia in Med. Chir. Rev. for July, 1834.

empty it, and the inflation may be repeated once or twice. It should not, I think, be done much oftener, and always with the greatest gentleness. The trachea pipe, which certain teachers have recommended to be carried by every accoucheur, should, in my opinion, never be resorted to.

EDITOR'S NOTE.

In cases of suspended animation at birth our treatment must be regulated by the cause of this condition. Thus, if the child's skin be blue, its lips and face livid and congested, a very few drops of blood allowed to escape from the cord may relieve the embarrassed circulation. But if, as more generally happens, the child be born in a state of syncope and anænia, friction with spirits over the chest, and still more so over the spine, the warm bath, alternated with cold aspersion in some cases, and either the Marshall Hall or Silvester methods of exciting respiration, which must be too familiar to the reader to need any description, should be at once resorted to and steadily persevered in for a long time. The Silvester method, with friction over the thorax and spine, and the warm bath, are the means I place most reliance on.—T. M. M.

S

OBSERVATIONS

ON CHLOROFORM.

SINCE the earlier edition of this work was published, the practice of inducing freedom from pain in surgical operations, in painful diseases, and in childbirth, by the inhalation of ethereal vapours, has been introduced into medicine. This process of Anæsthesia was at first effected by means of sulphuric ether, and considerable success followed the employment of that agent. Its utility in the practice of surgery led to its introduction into the lying-in room, and many women were saved the terrible pains of child-birth through its means. In the year 1848, another substance was suggested by Professor Simpson, of Edinburgh, as a substitute for ether. He was not satisfied that sulphuric ether was the best ingredient for producing anæsthesia; and after a long and laborious investigation of the properties of a great variety of fluids of the class of ethers, he came to the conclusion that Chloroform possesses various important advantages over them all, especially in obstetric practice; and that, in particular, it is far more

portable, more manageable and powerful, more
agreeable to inhale; is less exciting than ether, and
gives us far greater control and command over
the superinduction of the anæsthetic state. Dr.
Simpson's discovery of the valuable properties of
chloroform as an anæsthetic agent was followed
by its universal adoption. No other is employed
in surgery or midwifery; and although many
practitioners of eminence have not yet overcome
their scruples respecting the practice, yet a large
number have embraced the doctrine, that anæsthesia in midwifery is justifiable and safe. Indeed,
considering that eight years have not yet elapsed
since the promulgation of this discovery, the
number of its adherents is a matter of surprise,
particularly when we reflect upon the slowness
with which the greatest discoveries have been
received by mankind : witness the circulation of
the blood, and vaccination. When chloroform is
used to allay the pain of a surgical operation, it is
usual to carry its effects to the full amount of
insensibility. This is of great importance to the
operator as well as to the patient, for the sudden
movements, both voluntary and involuntary, which
most persons make when under the knife of the
surgeon, are thereby prevented, and the end is
accomplished with ease to both parties. Some
advocates for the employment of chloroform in
cases of parturition, recommend the effects to be

pushed to the same length as in surgical operations; but others are of opinion that the same amount of anæsthesia is not necessary, and that all the benefit of freedom from suffering in the pains of child-birth can be attained by a much more moderate use of this powerful agent. Dr. Murphy, Professor of Midwifery in the London University, and Dr. Beatty, Professor of Midwifery in the Royal College of Surgeons, Dublin, have both advocated this manner of employing chloroform in labour. They both recommend the use of the same instrument for the inhalation of the vapour. It is a small inhaler made by Coxeter, of London, a representation of which is given in Dr. Murphy's last work on chloroform, published in 1855. The great advantages of this instrument are the economy in the material to be used, the certainty that a sufficient quantity of atmospheric air is mixed with the chloroform vapour when passing into the lungs, the ease with which a patient can administer it to herself, and the security it affords against her taking too much. The latter is one of the most important advantages possessed by this method over every other. The vapour is in this way made its own protection against danger, for when a patient holds the inhaler in her own hand and applies it to her mouth, she continues to inspire as long as she is conscious, but the very moment she begins to lose consciousness, and long before any dangerous amount of chloroform could be taken, her hand drops, and the inhaler is thus removed from her mouth.

Dr. Fleming, of Dublin, has contrived and described an inhaler which is much used in surgical practice ; and, where the object is to produce and continue deep sopor, it answers remarkably well, but it could not be used in the way just spoken of in labour. Many practitioners continue to use the folded handkerchief, or a sponge, for the purpose of administering the chloroform, but these will probably adopt the method above described when they shall have made trial of it.

There are many points of importance to be attended to in the use of this powerful agent, viz. the quality of the drug; the time at which to commence its use ; the manner of using it ; and the dangers that attend it. *The quality of chloroform* is of the highest importance, for if it be not pure, some of those unpleasant effects spoken of by those who have used it in that condition will be produced. These are, severe cough and irritation of the bronchial mucous membrane, and excitement of the brain and nervous system, as evidenced by incoherent talking, violent efforts to get out of bed, &c. These effects are not produced when the drug is pure. The principal adulterations are alcohol and formic acid, which may be recognised by dropping some of the chloroform into a glass tube containing distilled water : it immediately sinks to the bottom; but, if impure, the globules assume a milky appearance, instead of remaining clear and bright.

The time at which to commence the use of chloroform in labour will depend upon the object aimed at by the attendant. If he is disposed to use it, as some do, only in cases requiring delivery by operation, of course the time will be regulated by that at which he feels himself called on to interfere with mechanical aid : but if he is inclined to employ this agent as a means of alleviating the pains of child-birth in ordinary cases, he must have some other rule to guide him. He should first decide whether the case is one in which he may safely make use of the drug; and it will be found that the cases forbidding it are very few indeed. With the exception of persons affected with disease of the heart, or brain, all others may be cautiously tested with chloroform, and when they are found to bear it well it may be persevered with. The time at which the trial is to begin will vary in different labours; no time can be fixed to suit all ; but it may be taken as a guide, that as the chloroform is employed to assuage pain, when that becomes urgent in any given case, that is the time to commence the inhalation of the anæsthetic. In the majority of cases this will be found to be about the time of the dilatation of the ós uteri, but in some first cases, when the os uteri is rigid and unyielding, the pains will be so violent and constant before the os uteri has yielded, that we will be compelled to administer chloroform during the first stage of labour, and sometimes· for some hours before it is terminated. When this is the case, it will be often found that the first stage is shortened by the treatment; the chloroform having the effect of relaxing the soft tissues, and favouring the natural dilatation of the parts. The time occupied in the administration will of course vary; sometimes, in women who have borne children before, half an hour will be all the time required, while in primiparæ, many hours, even up to ten, twelve, or fourteen, will be spent under the influence of the anæsthetic. This may be one reason for the disinclination exhibited by some practitioners to the use of this remedy; for it compels a close attendance in the sick-room after it is begun, and it is no doubt irksome to be thus confined, while in cases treated without chloroform a great portion of the time may be spent elsewhere. Such a motive should not weigh with any one really anxious for the welfare of his patient.

The mode of administration has been touched on already, when it was stated that for ordinary labours Coxeter's is the best contrivance. In whatever way the chloroform is used, the greatest caution is necessary in the beginning, for there is the greatest difference in the tolerance of different persons. Some (and particularly those of an hysterical temperament) are affected by the smallest quantity. Such a patient has been thrown into a state of insensibility, lasting for two hours, by the smell of a piece of lint that had been used with a liniment containing chloroform. Others (and they are the great majority) are more tolerant of the medicine, and require some time to bring them under its influence. It is well in all cases to begin by letting the patient smell the chloroform for a minute or two from the sponge in the chamber of the instrument; or, if a handkerchief be preferred, from a small quantity poured upon the corner of it. This cautionary proceeding serves to show whether there is any peculiar susceptibility in the patient, and also to accustom her to its odour. Having felt our way in this manner, and seen that small quantities do not produce any effects, we go on to measure the dose by allowing the patient to apply her mouth to the mouth-piece of the inhaler, or by bringing the handkerchief in a concave form over the mouth and nose. In whichever way we proceed, the quantity of chloroform should not at first exceed a teaspoonful. It is of the greatest importance that the system should be gradually brought under the anæsthetic influence: much of the danger, and most of the unpleasant effects, will be obviated by this course.

When the inhaler is used, it is necessary to be

sure that the patient does really inspire from it, for it will often be found that when she puts it to her mouth she shuts her lips and breathes through the nose alone. When this is perceived, she should be told to try to *suck* the fluid out of the instrument. By this manœuvre she will be taught to breathe through her mouth, and she will continue to do so. But sometimes it will be necessary to hold the nose, so as to compel her to breathe in the way desirable for our purpose.

When this course is pursued, the first effect usually perceived is the extinction of the terrible aching in the back, which, continuing between regular pains, is so distressing and induces the earnest demand for pressure on the back. This is removed, and the patient expresses the greatest relief and delight: very often she makes use of the phrase, ' This is heaven.' She knows when the pain is approaching, and calls for the chloroform: it may now be given to her again, and after the pain is over she will tell you she did not feel it near as much. In this way, without making her insensible, a vast amount of suffering is saved for many hours.

If the dose is made larger, or the inhalation is longer persevered in, a buzzing and reeling sensation in the head will be experienced : this speedily passes off when the chloroform is removed. If, on the contrary, it is persevered with, some incoherent talking may take place, the eyes will close, the limbs will fall, the hands will relax the grasp of the hand of the nurse or folded sheet, and anæsthetic sleep will follow. This having continued for a few moments, is succeeded by a happy consciousness of relief from pain. When a few of the usual pains have been thus treated, the patient may be allowed to use the inhaler herself, for from what has been just stated she cannot get too much; her hand will drop from her mouth as soon as she has taken enough to cause approaching sleep. The patient should be watched well at first, so as to ensure the action of the medicine to be such as described, for in some cases a spasmodic fixing of the muscles takes place about the time of the approach of insensibility; and in such a case the inhaler might be fixed tightly to the mouth, and the inhalation prolonged too far. When it is perceived that such an effect as this is not produced, the patient may be trusted to hold the instrument in her own hand. The chloroform must be renewed from time to time. The patient will complain that it is weak, and does her no good. When this occurs, it is well for the attendant to try it himself, and, finding the vapour deficient, he must pour in another charge. This will occur in ordinary first labours about eight times in the hour, so that we may say an ounce will be consumed every hour under ordinary circumstances. As delivery approaches, the quantity of chloroform may be increased, but it may be taken as a general rule that, with very few exceptions, no greater amount of effect will be required than that just described. Some cases will occur, in which the tolerance of the drug is so great, and the difficulty of overcoming the pain such, that the fuller effect must be produced, and the patient must be rendered insensible and kept so even for hours. In operations the deeper effects should be produced, for we thereby not only relieve all pain, but facilitate the operation by keeping the patient quiet.

The dangers of chloroform have been most marvellously magnified by some of the 'old school' practitioners; but experience shows every day more and more that a little familiarity with the medicine, and proper precaution in its use, are all that is necessary to ensure perfect safety in handling it.

That deaths have occurred under other circumstances, such as surgical operations, tooth-drawing, &c., cannot be denied, but it is a striking fact that in no instance of parturition is it recorded that death has been caused by the use of chloroform. The recumbent posture, and an empty stomach, are essential for the safe employment of chloroform. Both of these conditions are fulfilled in parturition, and unless gross neglect and mismanagement intervene, there is no likelihood of mischief taking place. If the rules above laid down be observed, it is almost impossible that anything unpleasant could occur.

The pains are sometimes suspended at first, when

the vapour is inhaled : they soon, however, return, and then, unless too great an effect is subsequently produced, they continue with regularity.

The tendency to hemorrhage after delivery is certainly increased by the use of the medicine, and therefore particular care must be observed, after the birth of the child, to guard against this very unpleasant consequence. In any case where hemorrhage has been known to have occurred after previous labours, the precaution of giving a full dose of ergot of rye, just as the child's head is passing through the vulva, should be adopted. This practice, as formerly recommended by Dr. Beatty, as a means of preventing hemorrhage in patients predisposed to it, will be found to be of great value in such cases when chloroform is employed.

The recovery after chloroform has been used is rapid and safe. It is observed that there is less of that great exhaustion that follows long and difficult labours. The nervous system has been saved to a great degree, and the vital energy of the patient not being diminished, she soon regains her former state of strength and health.

I am indebted for the matter of this chapter to my friend Dr. Thomas Beatty. The subject is one of which I have no personal knowledge—the use of chloroform having been introduced since my attention has been turned from medical practice.

CHAPTER XXIV.

ON THE MODERN TYPE AND TREATMENT OF PUERPERAL FEVER.

THE prevailing type of disease has undergone a complete alteration within the last quarter of a century. When this work was first published, the prevailing type of disease was stenic or inflammatory; at present it is asthenic or typhoid.

The true inflammatory form of puerperal fever now seldom occurs, and the disease, which is unfortunately more common than was formerly the case, generally assumes a low typhoid character. Indeed, the puerperal fever of the present day has so many points of analogy with erysipelas as to be considered by the most eminent modern authorities to be identical with that disease. The puerperal fever we now meet with presents all the symptoms of blood-poisoning, and is essentially a disease of debility. And hence the active antiphlogistic treatment and regimen, blood-letting, leeching, calomel and opium, and low diet formerly prescribed, are now seldom or never resorted to or required.

T

Under any circumstances the treatment of puerperal fever is most unsatisfactory. During the recent discussion on puerperal fever in the Dublin Obstetrical Society, Dr. Stokes thus communicated his great experience on this subject :— ' I have been a practising physician in Dublin for more than forty years. I have been repeatedly called in consultation to cases of puerperal fever in the better class of life, and I am sorry to say that the result is, that in these forty years I have never seen one case of puerperal fever in private practice that was not fatal—not one.' *

In our hospital practice, although the disease is generally fatal, yet I have seen several cases which have undoubtedly recovered from the worst form of puerperal fever. Unfortunately, however, these cases were but exceptions.

Nearly all the cases of puerperal fever which have come under my observation were of the typhoid or asthenic form of the disease. It is obvious that this does not admit of depletion, but urgently requires the free administration of stimulants and nutriment—brandy or wine, beef tea, chicken broth, jelly, arrowroot, &c., frequently repeated in small quantities at a

* Dublin Quarterly Journal of Medical Science, Aug. 1869, p. 313.

time, either by the mouth or by enemata, or through both channels.

The only drug on which I place much reliance in the treatment of puerperal fever is turpentine. This was first suggested many years ago by the late Dr. Brennan of Dublin, who incurred no small amount of ridicule for the suggestion. Turpentine appears to exercise a remarkable influence on this form of inflammation, and when it is tolerated by the stomach, which is not always the case, it generally relieves the distressing tympanitis, abdominal tenderness and pain better than any other medicine. The turpentine may be given in drachm doses and conjoined, or not as the symptoms may indicate, with small doses of opium as in the following formula, which is often prescribed in the Rotunda Hospital.

R Sp^ls Terebinthinæ Rect.   ℥i.
    Ætheris chlorici.   ℳx.
    Acetum Opii   ℳxv.
    Mucilaginis Acaciæ   ℥i.
    Aquæ Camphoræ   ℥i.
M. fiat Haust. to be repeated every fourth hour.

The turpentine may also be administered by enemeta if there be no diarrhea, and should be also sprinkled on the stupes that are necessary in every case of puerperal fever.

Turpentine cannot be given when there is either

vomiting or purging. The former symptom,
especially when the matter vomited has the
characteristic green or coffee-ground appearance,
is very unfavourable, and must be checked, if
possible, by small doses—one or two drops—of the
dilute hydrocyanic acid repeated every four or
five hours.

In such cases a small mustard sinapism may
be applied over the epigastrium; ice may be
administered, and milk and soda-water given as
a form of nutriment likely to be retained on the
stomach. If diarrhea supervenes, it must be
met by strong astringents, such as decoction of
logwood, with kino or catechu, or still better by
enemata such as this:—

> Tincturæ Opii   ℳxxv.
> Mucilaginis Amylæ   ʒi.
> M. fiat Enema.

I have seen a trial given to other medicines
recently advised—such as barm, the sulphites of
magnesia, soda, and potash, the chlorate of
potash, &c., but my experience of these remedies
does not lead me to dwell further on their use in
a work intended to teach the most approved
mode of practice, especially when treating of a
disease so serious as to afford no time for trying
therapeutic experiments.

In the inflammatory form of puerperal fever,

or true puerperal metro-peritonitis, occurring in
a woman of naturally strong constitution, which
form of the disease is now comparatively rarely
met with in practice, in addition to the remedies
already spoken of, which may also be used in this
as well as in the form of the disease more commonly met with, we may apply from twelve to
twenty-four leeches, as the case may be, over the
seat of pain, and thus afford great relief to the
patient's sufferings. In such cases, small alternative doses of grey powder and opium may be
cautiously administered, as for example :—

> ℞ Hydrargyri cum Creta   gr. ii.
> Sodæ Exiccatæ   gr. i.
> Pulv. Ipecacuanhæ co   gr. iii.
> M. fiat Pulv.: one every third hour.

The patient's strength must be supported, however, at the same time by beef tea, chicken broth,
or wine when required ; puerperal fever being
essentially a disease of debility.

In every case of puerperal fever, stupes and
poultices over the entire abdomen are required,
and the accoucheur should himself see that these
are properly employed, or only entrust this duty
to a very careful nurse. Great relief will generally be experienced from stuping the patient's
abdomen for some time with cloths wrung out
of hot water, sprinkled with turpentine, and ap-

plied as warm as they can be borne. The stuping must be followed by large hot poultices, covering the abdomen from the ensiform cartilage to the pubis, and repeated as long as any pain or tenderness remains.

CHAPTER XXV.

ON THE THIRD ORDER OF DIFFICULT LABOURS----
CRANIOTOMY AND CEPHALOTRIPSY.

THE third order of difficult labour includes all
cases of tedious labour in which the presentation
is natural, but in which the difficulty is so great
that it is considered necessary either to lessen
the bulk of the child, or else to provide for it a
passage larger than the natural one. The first
object may be accomplished by the use of instruments such as the perforator and crochet, the
cranioclast, and the cephalotribe, the use of
which is incompatible with the birth of a living
child. The second object may be attained by
the Cæsarean section, and according to some
authorities by the sigaultean operation, or division of the symphysis pubis.

The causes of the third order of difficult labours
are chiefly the various deformities to which the
pelvis is subject, whether resulting from rickets,
mollities ossium, congenital malformations of the
pelvis, or bony tumours. It may also be occasioned by diseases of the soft parts, intra-uterine

fibroid, and other tumours, ovarian and vaginal tumours, cicatrices, contractions and occlusions of the os uteri and vagina. The fœtus may be so malformed or disproportioned that it cannot pass through the natural passages, and this may result from simple disproportion, the fœtus being very large or the passages very small, or from either maternal or fœtal deformity or disease.

The various malformations of the pelvis, and the mode of diagnosing them, have been explained in the first chapter of this work.

In these cases, if consulted sufficiently early, we have to choose between those operations by which the child is certainly destroyed to afford a better chance of safety to the mother, and those by which a chance of life is afforded to both. It is obvious that no more serious and important problem can be entertained, involving, as this does, the life or death of one if not two individuals, whose fate hangs on the judgment and determination of the accoucheur in such cases.

The rule of British midwifery practice is that laid down in the last edition of this work (p. 135), and expressed in almost similar terms by nearly all the other standard British obstetric writers— i.e. that 'our reasons for operating should be drawn entirely from the state of the mother, which ought also to determine our choice of instruments,' the paramount consideration in such cases being the safety of the mother, to which, in accordance with this rule, everything else must be sacrificed.

The cases in which craniotomy is required is a subject on which much difference of opinion exists ; and I shall therefore, in the first instance, quote the rules approved of by the majority of British obstetric writers, such as Dr. Churchill, Dr. Maunsell, Dr. Ramsbotham, Dr. Meadows, and Dr. Barnes, and then give my own views on this subject, and my reasons for dissenting from those of such eminent authorities.

According to the above-named writers, craniotomy is required when the pelvis is so deformed that the narrowest diameter at the brim or outlet is less than two inches and three quarters, or three inches. 2nd. If the child be hydrocephalic to such an extent that the head cannot pass through a normal pelvis. 3rd. Where the child is so wedged in by two or more parts presenting, that it cannot be extracted by the forceps. 4th. In some cases of great flooding before delivery, in which the forceps cannot be applied. 5th. In similar cases of convulsion, rupture of the uterus, and other varieties of complex labour. 6th. Where the pelvis is so occupied by tumours as to prevent the passage of the child. 7th. When the child is dead and the labour protracted.

For my own part, I can only agree with the

last of these rules, namely, that craniotomy is required in cases of very protracted labour when the child is dead, to save the mother from the serious ill consequences of tedious labour. In all the other cases we are, I think, bound to consider duly the comparative advantages offered by other operations, such as version as a substitute for craniotomy, the application of the long forceps, hysterotomy and the induction of premature labour, as compared with craniotomy.

Craniotomy is an operation which should be only regarded as a measure of necessity, and never as one of election. That is to say, that whenever delivery may be otherwise accomplished, craniotomy should not be thought of. The cases in which this cruel operation is required are very few and far between. Thus in my own practice, before and since my connection with the largest Lying-in Hospital in Great Britain, I have never performed on a living child, what Dr. Radford has described as ' that dreadful expedient, nay, shall I not call it murderous operation, craniotomy.' *

The late Sir James Simpson thus expresses himself on this subject. He says—' Formerly medical practitioners seem to have thought little, and medical writers said little, regarding the

---

* Radford on the Cæsarean Section, &c., p. 64.

very repulsive and revolting character of craniotomy when performed, as it frequently was, when
the child was still living. . . . But, perhaps, ere
long, it will become a question in professional
ethics, whether a professional man is, under the
name of a so-called operation, justified in deliberately destroying the life of a living human
being.'

Craniotomy is thus performed:—the patient
being placed in the ordinary obstetric position,
and her bladder and rectum being previously
emptied, the operator introduces two fingers of
his left hand into the vagina up to the child's
head; guided and protected by these, so as to
avoid injuring the soft parts, the perforator is
then introduced by the accoucheur's right hand
up to the point of the head that presents, into
which it is inserted till the skull be pierced.
The blades are then pushed in as far as their
shoulders, and the handles are forcibly separated
by an assistant—at first in the position in which
they were originally placed, and again at right
angles to this, so as to make a crucial opening,
through which the brain, which is broken up by
pushing the instrument in all directions through
the cerebral structure, may escape. It is generally recommended that some time should now
elapse, to allow the skull to collapse, after which
the crochet is to be passed in with the same pre-

caution as the perforator, and being fixed on the edge of the perforated bone, the operator's fingers acting as a *point d'appui* on the opposite side of it, to prevent slipping and laceration, the head is to be drawn down by force in the direction of the axis of the pelvis.

The dangers of craniotomy are many and great. In the first place, the perforator, or crochet, may slip on the way to the head of the child, or from it, and may lacerate the vagina or uterus. Secondly, the perforator has been known, as Dr. Barnes says, ' to strike the promontory of the sacrum, or lacerate the cervix uteri. Thirdly, spicula of cranial bones resulting from perforation may scratch or tear the soft parts.' Fourthly, the shock inflicted on the patient's nervous system is greater and more lasting in its effects than when the forceps, or version, have been resorted to. Fifthly, inflammation of the uterus, or vagina, is a not unfrequent sequence of craniotomy.

The mortality to the mother, for whose sake the child is often sacrificed, in craniotomy cases is higher than is the case when any other recognised midwifery operation, with the exception of the Cæsarean section, is performed. This has been conclusively proved by Dr. Churchill's admirably arranged statistics, by which it appears that in eight hundred craniotomy cases, one hundred and forty-one of the mothers, or almost one in five and a half, were lost. If we compare this with the result of any of the obstetric operations by which it is attempted to save both mother and child, we find that the mortality in craniotomy cases is much more unfavourable to the mother than it is in those cases which are delivered by version, the long forceps, or the induction of premature labour.

The cephalotribe is a pair of forceps of great length and strength, the blades of which can be very forcibly and closely approximated together by means of a screw placed in the handle. The object of this instrument is to compress and crush down the fœtal skull after perforation has been effected. The cephalotribe was invented by M. Baudeloque, and has since been variously modified by the late Sir James Simpson, Dr. Kidd of Dublin, Dr. Braxton Hicks, and others.

A new mode of performing embryotomy in cases of extreme pelvic deformity, by means of Weisse's Ecraseur, was recently demonstrated before the Obstetrical Society of London by Dr. Barnes. But as I am not aware that this operation has been carried into practice, I need not dwell on the mode of performing it.

CHAPTER XXVI.

ON THE CÆSAREAN OPERATION.

IN British midwifery practice the Cæsarean section is so rarely performed that few English practitioners have any opportunity of witnessing it. Thus in the largest obstetric institution in this country, the Rotunda Hospital, but one case of the Cæsarean operation has occurred from its foundation in 1757 to the present time.

Therefore, as two cases of this kind have come under my observation, in one of which I operated myself, I venture to speak with more confidence on the subject than I would otherwise do. The statistics of this operation show that rather less than one half of the patients operated on recover, and that about three-fourths of the number of children are extracted alive. In this country the mortality occasioned by the Cæsarean section is far higher than it is on the Continent. The reason of this is that the operation is not resorted to here till all other means having failed, and the patient being exhausted by a tedious and painful labour, the Cæsarean section is performed as the *dernier recours* of the practitioner, and the last chance of the mother. The only wonder is that an operation performed under such unfavourable circumstances should have succeeded even as often as it has done. Dr. Churchill, with his wonted research, has collected out of the records of British and American practice eighty cases of hysterotomy, in which twenty-three mothers were saved and fifty-seven lost, or more than two-thirds. In seventy-seven of these cases the result to the child is thus stated, forty-four were saved and thirty-three were lost, or nearly one-half.

In foreign practice, where the operation is resorted to under more favourable conditions, the results are more successful. Thus M. Duffeillay collected the cases which are recorded from 1858 to 1864, and states that in these cases there had been seventy-five per cent. of recoveries. This must be confessed, however, to be far more favourable than the results reported by any other writer. Dr. Churchill, for example, has collected from foreign authorities a large number of cases, the result of which was that one-half of the total number proved fatal to the mothers, and one-third of the children extracted were still-born.

In several instances the Cæsarean section has been repeatedly performed on the same patient; and one case is recorded in which this operation was repeated seven times on the same woman by her own husband !

The most frequent cause of the Cæsarean section is extreme deformity of the pelvis, resulting from mollities ossium, or rickets.

Dr. Radford * has collected the history of seventy-seven cases, in which the Cæsarean section has been performed in Great Britain. In these cases the operation was caused by mollities ossium in forty-three instances; by rickets in fourteen; by fibrous or other tumours in the pelvis in six; by congenital distortion of the pelvis in one; by an exostosis from the sacrum in two; by fracture of the pelvis in two; by carcinoma of the os and cervix uteri in two; and in seven cases the cause which led to the performance of the Cæsarean section is not recorded.

The rule approved of by the majority of British obstetricians is, that the Cæsarean section is justified only when the pelvis is so contracted that a dead or mutilated child cannot be delivered per *vias naturales* with safety to the mother. This rule, as will be seen in the following remarks, I do not coincide with.

In several of the reported British cases of hysterotomy, the operation was not resorted to until embryotomy had been first performed and failed,

* 'Observations on the Cæsarean Section and other Obstetric Operations.' By Thomas Radford, M.D., p. 4. Manchester: 1865.

owing to the pelvis being so deformed that it was found impossible to drag the fœtus, even after mutilation, through it. Under these circumstances the Cæsarean section has been performed, for no practitioner would suffer a patient to die undelivered with a mutilated fœtus still in utero. But would not the patient have been afforded a far better chance of safety, if the living child had been extracted by the Cæsarean section, without subjecting the mother to the additional risk of craniotomy, as well as the protracted suffering and danger of tedious labour?

I do not here speak of the morality in such a case, of destroying an unborn child which might have been possibly extracted alive by the Cæsarean section, with a fair chance of safety to its mother. This point is one on which I have always entertained, and have not hesitated to express, a very strong opinion. I do not believe that we are morally justified in destroying either mother or child for any purpose. But this topic is not one to be discussed in a work such as this. I have therefore merely expressed my own opinion, as well as given that generally held and acted on in this country.

Extensive malignant disease of the os or cervix uteri, so situated as to prevent its dilatation during labour, has in some instances required and led to the performance of the Cæsarean section. In cases of extra-uterine fœtation, where there is danger to the mother's life from the bursting of the cyst containing the fœtus, when pregnancy is sufficiently advanced, this operation has been recommended. It has also been advised in some cases of rupture of the uterus occurring during labour, and in cases of rapidly developing malignant disease, especially if attended with much hemorrhage, or where the disease is rapidly undermining the patient's health and enfeebling the fœtus.

The Cæsarean section should be resorted to immediately after death, if a pregnant woman dies undelivered, for the purpose of rescuing the child. The child in utero. may, in cases of sudden death from violence or disease, survive its mother much longer than is sometimes supposed; or, as Dr. Burns expresses it,—'The uterus may live longer than the body, and after the mother has been quite dead, the child still continues its functions.' This is borne out by analogy; for in some of the lower animals it has been proved that the fœtus will live separately for some time if the membranes be unruptured. Harvey says:—'Children have been frequently taken out of the womb alive hours after the death of the mother.' Dr. Jackson recovered an infant half-an-hour after the death of the mother. I have myself failed to resuscitate the child in a case in which I extracted it by the Cæsarean section within fifteen minutes after the mother's death. There can be no doubt, however, of the fact that living children have been thus ex- tracted a considerable time after the mother's death ; and it is therefore our duty, whenever a pregnant mother dies undelivered, to afford this chance of life to the child.

With regard to the best period of pregnancy, I perfectly agree with Dr. Greenhalgh's obser- vation at the Dublin meeting of the British Medical Association, namely, that ' greater success would attend our endeavours if all cases were operated upon at or shortly after the com- pletion of the eighth month of utero-gestation, when the vessels are smaller, the contractile power of the uterus greater, and the liquor amnii relatively greater in proportion to the size of the child. . . . A smaller incision would then be required, less blood would be lost, and the ex- traction of the fœtus would be greatly facili- tated.'* If the operation be deferred till labour has set in, it should at any rate, if possible, be performed before the rupture of the membranes.

The Cæsarean section is performed in the fol- lowing manner :—The temperature of the patient's room must be raised to about 78° or 80°, and,

* British Medical Journal, Dec. 7, 1867, p. 518.

her rectum and bladder being emptied, she is to be placed on a hard mattress, lying on her back. Whether chloroform should be administered or not in these cases is a disputed question, and depends on circumstances. The operation is not a very painful one, and it is important to avoid exciting vomiting, which chloroform sometimes does. On the other hand, the shock to the patient's nervous system may be diminished, and the operation facilitated, by chloroform in some of these cases. A careful stethescopic examination must be made to ascertain the situation of the placenta, which is to be avoided.

The operation consists in a bold incision eight or ten inches in length extending along the linea alba from below the umbilicus to a short distance above the pubis. Great care must be taken not to wound the bladder or cut through the umbilicus by this incision. The first incision should be made through the integuments, fascia, and tendon of the linea alba, and not wound the peritoneum, which should be carefully divided on a director. The uterus will now be exposed, and is to be laid open by rapidly, but carefully, dividing its muscular tissue in the situation of the body, avoiding the fundus and cervix uteri, as well as the situation of the placenta, in so doing. The incision through the uterus, which is to be somewhat shorter than that through the abdominal parietes, will expose the membranes. These must be ruptured, and the liquor amnii taken up by the sponges which the assistants have in readiness for the purpose, while the operator introduces his hand through the wound, seizes the child by the feet, and extracts it as quickly as possible, great care and promptitude being necessary to prevent the neck of the fœtus being caught by the contracting edges of the uterine wound. The placenta and membranes must be then immediately removed, and a small probang or elastic catheter passed down through the os uteri to clear the passage for the escape of the discharges.

No sutures are required in the uterus, as this organ rapidly contracts after the extraction of the child, and thus diminishes the size of the incision to a mere slit, which in favourable cases soon unites.

Before closing the external wound, if any hemorrhage or escape of liquor amnii has taken place into the abdominal cavity, it should be lightly and rapidly sponged out by the assistants. The edges of the wound may now be brought together. This is generally done by means of interrupted silver sutures, which are sometimes recommended to be passed through the peritoneum as well as the abdominal parietes, so as to ensure the union of the former membrane; or by means of the uninterrupted silk suture, which Dr. Spencer Wells used with success in one case. The great point is to secure the *complete* closure of the wound.   This should be assisted by straps of adhesive plaster between and above the sutures, and over all this either cold water, or, perhaps, Lister's carbolic dressing should be placed.

The duties of the assistants, of whom there should be two at hand, as well as an experienced nurse, are almost as important as those of the operator during the performance of the Cæsarean section.   Their chief business is to prevent the extrusion of the intestines by guarding them *in situ* by warm flannels over the exposed abdominal cavity, and afterwards to prevent their strangulation in the uterine wound, or during the approximation of the abdominal incision, and to restrain hemorrhage on the escape of the liquor amnii into the peritoneal cavity.

The after treatment is most important to attend to, as some of the deaths after the Cæsarean section have resulted from neglecting this rather than from the operation itself.   Immediately after the operation a full opiate should be given, and this may be generally best administered in a little brandy.   Vomiting should be at once checked by diluted hydrocyanic acid, creasote, and ice.   After some hours the patient's strength may be supported by a little chicken broth or other light nourishment. The most perfect quiet of mind and body must be maintained for many days. When death occurs in these cases, it may be caused by shock, hemorrhage, exhaustion, or from peritonitis, for all of which the practitioner must be on the watch until the patient is quite convalescent.

CHAPTER XXVII.

ON VERSION AS A SUBSTITUTE FOR CRANIOTOMY OR
THE LONG FORCEPS.

THE practice of turning in some cases of contracted pelvis was revived a few years ago on the
authority of the late Sir James Simpson. This
idea, however, I believe first originated with an
· Irish accoucheur, Sir Fielding Ould, the second
Master of the Rotunda Hospital, whose views on
this subject, published in his ' Practice of Midwifery,' in 1742, are almost identical with those
now enforced.

The cases of head presentation, in which version is recommended by Dr. Barnes and other
recent writers, are cases of difficult labour arising
from slight disproportion between the passage
and the body to be propelled through it, and
caused by pelvic contraction, or by the fœtal
head being larger or more firmly ossified than
usual.

The grounds on which turning is recommended
in such cases in preference to the long forceps,

or craniotomy, are thus stated : The base of the skull is narrower than the inter-parietal diameter, and the head is more compressible under tractile than under expulsive efforts ; or, as otherwise expressed, the head will pass through the strait of the pelvis more easily when the base comes first than when the vertex comes first. Another and a very important reason for this operation is, that it may be attempted at a much earlier period of labour than craniotomy, and therefore affords the mother a better chance of safety.

Some eminent obstetricians do not coincide with these views. The weight of modern as well as former authority is, I think, in favour of the operation of turning, under the circumstances already referred to. The risk to the mother is not increased by this operation, when properly and judiciously performed ; and with regard to the child, as Dr. Barnes says : 'It is enough to justify the operation if we save a child now and then. I believe, however, that exercising reasonable care in selection of cases, and skill in execution, more than one-half the children may be saved ; and to save even one child out of twenty is something to set off against the deliberate sacrifice of all.' *

* 'Lectures on Obstetric Operations,' by Robert Barnes, M.D. London, 1870, p. 276.

I have myself performed version as a substitute for the application of the long forceps in six cases. Four of the children so delivered were born alive, and five of the mothers recovered, one dying of puerperal fever, which, however, was prevalent at the time.

CHAPTER XXVIII.

ON THE INDUCTION OF PREMATURE LABOUR.

THE induction of premature labour *for the purpose of saving both mother and child* from some grave risk, which would be imminent to either if gestation went on to its full period, has only lately come to be justly regarded as a legitimate, and in certain cases most valuable, obstetric operation.

This operation affords us what must be regarded as the greatest desideratum in midwifery, namely, a substitute, in fitting cases, for both craniotomy and the Cæsarean section.

In the year 1756, we learn from Denman, that a meeting of obstetricians was held in London, for the purpose of discussing the propriety of this operation, and at which its performance was sanctioned. Shortly afterwards it was performed with success by Dr. Macaulay and Dr. Kelly, the latter of whom operated thus three times in successive pregnancies on the same patient. Still the operation met with great opposition in France as well as in England, and has not until very lately been fully approved of in this country.

The induction of premature labour would be a criminal offence if attempted before the period at which the fœtus is viable; that is, as a rule, before the completion of the seventh month of pregnancy, or for any purpose but that of saving the lives of both mother and child under the circumstances just referred to.

This operation is justifiable in the following cases: first, where such an amount of pelvic deformity or disease exists as to prevent the safe passage of a full-grown fœtus, but in which a viable fœtus may nevertheless pass through the pelvis; secondly, in cases in which, as sometimes happens, the fœtus perishes in successive pregnancies at a certain period of utero-gestation, at which extra-uterine life is possible; thirdly, in some cases in which at the same period the pregnancy is complicated by convulsions, cancer, or fibrous tumours of the uterus, incontrollable vomiting, serous effusions into the pleura or peritoneal cavities resulting from pregnancy, rupture of the uterus in previous labours, and great ante-partum hemorrhage. All these and some other cases, under certain circumstances, for a full consideration of which I would refer more particularly to the writings of Dr. Churchill and Dr. Barnes on this subject, have led to and justified the induction of premature labour as soon as the fœtus was viable.

The means by which premature labour may be induced are chiefly mechanical, as all the drugs which were supposed to be effectual in this way are either useless and uncertain, or dangerous to mother and child. The other agents resorted to for this purpose all act on the uterus by exciting reflex nervous action.

No practitioner should ever undertake the responsibility of inducing premature labour on himself. This operation should always be first sanctioned by a full and deliberate consultation of the best practitioners whose advice can be obtained.

Rupture of the membranes was until of late years the only mode of inducing premature labour, and it still remains a certain, and perhaps the safest, means of effecting this object. The best way of performing this operation is that recommended by Hopkins many years ago, i. e., 'to pass the hand some distance between the ovum and the uterine walls, and then to tap the amniotic sac at a point distant from the os. By this mode it was sought to provide for the gradual escape of the liquor amnii.' The direct rupture of the membranes may also be accomplished by the passage of an ordinary gum elastic catheter, with half an inch of the top cut off, through the os uteri just into the uterus, and then passing the stillet through the catheter so as to puncture the membranes, and allow the liquor amnii to drain away.

A very effectual but very dangerous method of inducing premature labour is the intra-uterine douche, first proposed by a German writer in 1825, and thirty years afterwards again brought into notice by the late Sir James Simpson, and modified and improved on by Dr. Sinclair, of Dublin, who has devised a very effectual double-cylinder syringe for this purpose. The operation consists in throwing alternate streams of cold and tepid water against the os uteri by a vaginal syringe; this may be continued for about ten minutes at a time, and repeated at long intervals till the desired effect be produced. This generally takes place after the third or fourth douche: but in one case, related in Drs. Johnston and Sinclair's ' Practical Midwifery,' labour did not set in until after the application of fifteen douches.

The vaginal, and especially the intra-uterine douche, however cautiously they may be used for the purpose of inducing premature labour, are always hazardous and attended by great danger of causing the mother's death. In such cases the cause of death is generally the entrance of air into the uterine sinuses, or, according to Dr. Churchill, of fluid into the peritoneal cavity through the Fallopian tubes. A fatal case of this kind came under my own observation about two years ago, and would make me hesitate very much before again taking part in this operation with the intra-uterine douche.

The separation of the membranes for two or three inches round the os, either by the finger or a soft flexible bougie passed through the os, has been recommended by several eminent authorities for this purpose. The dilatation of the os uteri by sponge tents was also resorted to, amongst others by the late Sir James Simpson. Dr. Barnes prefers to effect the dilatation of the cervix uteri by a peculiarly formed elastic ' fiddle-shaped' bag, which is introduced into the cervical canal and dilated until the cervix will admit three or four fingers, after which the membranes are ruptured and the dilator again employed until the parts are sufficiently expanded to admit of the birth of the child. A necessary preliminary to Dr. Barnes' operation is the introduction of a piece of elastic bougie into the uterus, between it and the membranes; this is suffered to remain *in situ* for several hours before the second part of the operation is undertaken.

CHAPTER XXIX.

ON INVERSION OF THE UTERUS.

INVERSION of the uterus is one of the rarest and most dangerous complications of labour. Thus, in the Dublin Lying-in Hospital but one case of this kind has occurred, although over 192,000 women have been delivered in the institution.

Inversion of the uterus may be either acute or chronic. In the following remarks we shall confine ourselves to the consideration of the former. The term acute inversion of the uterus is limited to those cases of this accident which are of recent occurrence and which come under our notice immediately after their occurrence, or at least during the period within which the physiological changes which take place in the uterus after parturition are still going on. Subsequently to this period the case becomes one of chronic inversion.

There are three distinct forms or rather degrees of inversion of the uterus. In the first there is merely a cup-shaped depression of that portion of the fundus to which the placenta was attached. In the second, this depression is converted into a regular intussusception of the upper portion of the uterus, which is forced down towards the os. The third variety of this accident is complete inversion, the fundus and body of the uterus being completely displaced pass through the cervix and os, which in extreme cases is also turned inside out, and protrude from the vulva.

Inversion of the uterus may result from morbid growths within the womb, as well as a complication of parturition. The latter is, however, seven times more frequent than the former.

The most frequent cause of inversion of the womb is unskilful management of the third stage of labour; the uterus being inverted in fully nine-tenths of all the cases recorded of this accident by undue traction on the cord, or excessive pressure over the fundus, but most generally by forcible traction on the funis, to hasten the expulsion of the placenta.

It is important to bear in mind that inversion of the uterus may take place spontaneously and quite irrespective of any malpractice. These cases are exceeding rare.

In some instances on record this accident appears to have been produced by other causes besides that just mentioned, as for example, by shortness of the funis, by the pelvis being abnormally capacious, by delivery taking place when the patient was in the erect position, by precipitate labour, by the patient making extraordinary expulsive efforts to force off the placenta. These causes and others have been assigned for some of the published cases of this kind. But, after all, the fact is indisputable that the usual cause of inversion of the uterus is improper traction on the funis in the third stage of labour, the placenta being still adherent to the uterus.

As the accident is fortunately so rarely met with in Dublin midwifery practice I shall make no apology for giving the following abridgment of a case I recently published in a monograph on this subject. Some months ago whilst lecturing at the hospital (May 19, 1870), I was sent for by a medical practitioner to assist him in a labour case. On my arrival, within a few minutes, I found the patient in a state of collapse, pulseless, icy cold, blanched, respiration sighing, and exhibiting all the symptoms which generally attend cases of great hemorrhage. That this had taken place was evinced by the saturated condition of the patient's bed. The uterus was completely inverted, and was protruding between her legs, with the placenta firmly adherent to the fundus, from which a considerable draining of blood was still going.

The history of the case was as follows:—The

patient, a young woman aged eighteen, who had been married in her fifteenth year, was delivered of her third child that afternoon at a quarter past four o'clock. She had a very quick and easy labour, although the membranes ruptured early. After the birth of the child there was considerable hemorrhage during the third stage. The midwife endeavoured to press the placenta off, and failing to do so, introduced two fingers into the os to ascertain, as she stated, if the placenta was adherent or not; directing another woman meanwhile to make firm pressure over the fundus uteri. She denied making any traction on the cord at this moment, when, suddenly, and as she alleged from the pressure over the fundus, the womb became completely inverted and was extruded from the vulva. Dr. Torney was now called in, and on his arrival, finding the woman pulseless and considering the serious nature of the case, sent up to the hospital for further assistance, and, in the meantime, very judiciously administered stimulants and applied a sinapism over the heart.

When I arrived the woman was in the condition just described, and accordingly, having first administered as large a quantity of brandy and ammonia as I could get her to swallow, I at once proceeded to peel off the placenta which was morbidly adherent to a great part of the fundus.

She was lying in a pool of blood when I examined her, and the hemorrhage was going on to a considerable extent before and during the operation, but was not increased by it. On the contrary, it stopped almost immediately after it. I then returned the uterus, still inverted, completely within the vagina; the part that extruded last being the first returned, and applying pressure steadily to the fundus, with great difficulty succeeded in pushing it through the inverted cervix, there being a persistent convexity of the fundus uteri which it took some time to overcome. I now had the satisfaction of feeling the uterus spring out back into the pelvis before my hand and resume its normal condition. Dr. Torney also introduced his hand and found the parts in their natural situation. We gave twenty drops of Battley's Liquor Opii with aromatic spirits of ammonia. She was still cold as death, jactitating, colourless and pulseless. I should now have at once resorted to transfusion, as the last and only hope of saving the patient's life. But, unfortunately, the circumstances of the case were such as to render this operation impossible, there being no one at hand to furnish the vital fluid to be injected, nor was there the necessary apparatus at our command, and hence, most reluctantly, I was obliged to abandon the idea of transfusion.

We applied fresh mustard sinapisms over the heart and to the calves of the legs, and hot jars were put to the feet. There was now hardly any draining from the vulva, and we bound her up and applied a large compress over the uterus, which was firmly contracted. The brandy and ammonia was administered by the spoonful every few minutes. Her head was lowered, and finding the vital powers still failing, we again gave thirty drops of Battley's Liquor Opii in some brandy with ammonia. Despite all our efforts, however, she sank rapidly and died before seven o'clock in the afternoon.

The symptoms of inversion of the uterus are always of a very grave and alarming character. Amongst them, the most constant and most prominent are the occurrence of a sudden and intense bearing-down pain in the womb at the moment the accident takes place. This is, almost invariably, immediately followed by a feeling of faintness and exhaustion, and the setting in of sudden collapse. The pulse becomes rapid, weak, and intermittent; the skin is cold and clammy, vomiting or nausea is complained of, the respiration is hurried and sighing, the patient tosses about moaning continually, and soon becomes unconscious. These symptoms are, of course, all aggravated by the profuse hemorrhage which generally attends inversion, and which is said to be greater in cases of partial than in complete inversion of the uterus. Cases of this kind accompanied by collapse have, however, been recorded in which little or no hemorrhage was observed. On examining the parts, if the inversion be complete, the nature of the case will be evident; but if it be only partial, or in the second degree, we must institute a vaginal examination, when a tumour will be found in the pelvis. This tumour will be globular in form, dipping down into a cul de sac about an inch or more in depth, within the os uteri.

If the case be one of simple depression of the fundus, the first degree of inversion, it will not be possible to reach the inverted part without introducing the hand within the uterus. But here we must, as in all these cases, examine with the hand above the pubis, when, if the case be one of complete inversion, or even of extreme introversion, we shall not find the hard, contracted uterine tumour in the natural position; and, if the case be one of depression of the fundus, we shall be able to trace the outline of the depressed part by an examination through the abdominal parietes.

Though it would be almost impossible that complete inversion could be overlooked; yet, it is by no means impossible that partial inversion might not be at once recognised. Hence, if a patient after delivery complains of sudden, intense bearing-down pain, or evinces symptoms of collapse and shock, not to be accounted for by any form of hemorrhage, the practitioner should bear in mind the possibility of the case being one of inversion, and at once institute a vaginal and abdominal examination; and if he does not find the globular fundus uteri in its normal position, or if he discover any tumour projecting into the vagina, he should consider and treat the case as one of partial inversion.

In the treatment of inversion of the uterus success or failure is mainly determined by the promptitude of the accoucheur in effecting the reduction of the displaced organ. For if this be postponed sufficiently long to allow the uterus to contract completely, replacement will be impossible, and the patient will either perish at once from hemorrhage and shock, or survive, the victim of the most distressing uterine suffering.

The difficulty of replacing a completely inverted uterus results from the constriction of the inverted part of the cervix. Every hour that elapses before replacement is attempted greatly increases the tumefaction of the protruded organ, and the pressure of the neck of the uterus, through which it must pass, until reduction

through the undilated cervix becomes imprac-
ticable. The case is now closely analogous to one
of strangulated hernia.

Denman found it impossible to replace an
inverted uterus four hours after the accident.

The question of removing the placenta, or not
removing it, before attempting the replacement
of the inverted uterus is one on which the opinions of obstetricians are almost equally divided.
Our limits do not enable us to consider the argu-
ments which are adduced in favour of either
practice.

Amongst Dublin obstetricians the weight of
authority is in favour of removing the placenta,
if adherent, before attempting to reduce the inverted uterus. Dr. Johnston, by his example and
precept, strongly supported this practice, which
is also advocated by the most eminent Irish
midwifery authorities; as for instance, by Dr.
Churchill, Dr. McClintock, Dr. Denham, and
others no less distinguished. Independent of all
authorities, however, the Dublin practice in such
cases has, I think, the weight of common sense
to support it.

In attempting to return the inverted uterus
to its natural situation, the part last protruded
through the cervix must be that first replaced.
In doing this, it is always essential to bear in
mind the direction of the axes of the pelvis, and

to press the uterus at first upwards and backwards into the hollow of the sacrum, and then upwards and forwards through the brim, in such a direction laterally as to avoid the promontory of the sacrum.

The mode of effecting the reduction of the displaced uterus, although the subject of much controversy, is in reality simple enough. The placenta, if adherent, having been quickly detached, the displaced uterus is to be grasped in the operator's right hand and pushed gently but firmly, *in globo*, into the vagina, the cervix being first returned. No attempt to replace the uterus should be made until the organ is fairly within the vagina, as otherwise a double inversion would be produced. When the uterus has been pushed as far within the vagina as possible, steady pressure should be made with the pulp of the fingers within the vagina on the fundus, which should thus be pressed through the cervix. Great caution is required in this operation to prevent the pressure exceeding the resisting powers of the uterine walls, or else a fatal laceration of the fundus might easily be, and indeed has been, thus produced. In this way the fundus should be insinuated back through the cervix, when pressure with the operator's knuckles may be substituted for the fingers, and continued until, as generally happens, the uterus will be found to spring out of itself, upwards and forwards, ' like a bottle of india-rubber when turned inside out,' as Dr. Churchill says, and thus the womb resumes its natural situation. The operator's hand should still, however, be kept in the uterus until, as occurred in the case narrated in this chapter, the organ is found to have contracted firmly, when it may be withdrawn. The after treatment must now be conducted on those general principles, already explained, which are applicable to all cases in which much hemorrhage and a great shock has been sustained by a parturient woman.

If the inverted uterus cannot be replaced after our efforts have been carried as far as is compatible with the patient's safety, the uterus should be at least pushed up within the vulva; hemorrhage must be restrained by astringent applications; inflammation should be met by appropriate treatment; the state of the bladder carefully attended to, and the pressure taken off the part as far as possible by properly adjusted bandages or pessaries. The further treatment of the case under these circumstances is not a question for consideration in a treatise on midwifery, as the case is now one of chronic inversion of the uterus, a subject which will be more properly discussed in a work on the diseases of women.

INDEX.

THE END.

LONDON: PRINTED BY
SPOTTISWOODE AND CO., NEW-STREET SQUARE
AND PARLIAMENT STREET

[MARCH 1872.]

GENERAL LIST OF WORKS

PUBLISHED BY

MESSRS. LONGMANS, GREEN, AND CO.

PATERNOSTER ROW, LONDON.

History, Politics, Historical Memoirs, &c.

The **HISTORY of ENGLAND** from the Fall of Wolsey to the Defeat of the Spanish Armada. By JAMES ANTHONY FROUDE, M.A. late Fellow of Exeter College, Oxford.
LIBRARY EDITION, 12 VOLS. 8vo. price £8 18s.
CABINET EDITION, in 12 vols. crown 8vo. price 72s.

The **HISTORY of ENGLAND** from the Accession of James II. By Lord MACAULAY.
STUDENT'S EDITION, 2 vols. crown 8vo. 12s.
PEOPLE'S EDITION, 4 vols. crown 8vo. 16s.
CABINET EDITION, 8 vols. post 8vo. 48s.
LIBRARY EDITION, 5 vols. 8vo. £4.

LORD MACAULAY'S WORKS. Complete and Uniform Library Edition. Edited by his Sister, Lady TREVELYAN. 8 vols. 8vo. with Portrait, price £5 5s. cloth, or £8 8s. bound in tree-calf by Rivière.

VARIETIES of VICE-REGAL LIFE. By Sir WILLIAM DENISON, K.C.B. late Governor-General of the Australian Colonies, and Governor of Madras. With Two Maps. 2 vols. 8vo. 28s.

On **PARLIAMENTARY GOVERNMENT in ENGLAND**; its Origin, Development, and Practical Operation. By ALPHEUS TODD, Librarian of the Legislative Assembly of Canada. 2 vols. 8vo. price £1 17s.

A **HISTORICAL ACCOUNT of the NEUTRALITY of GREAT BRITAIN DURING the AMERICAN CIVIL WAR.** By MOUNTAGUE BERNARD, M.A. Chichele Professor of International Law and Diplomacy in the University of Oxford. Royal 8vo. 16s.

The **CONSTITUTIONAL HISTORY of ENGLAND, since the Accession of George III. 1760—1860.** By Sir THOMAS ERSKINE MAY, C.B. Second Edition. Cabinet Edition, thoroughly revised. 3 vols. crown 8vo. price 18s.

The **HISTORY of ENGLAND, from the Earliest Times to the Year 1865.** By C. D. YONGE, B.A. Regius Professor of Modern History in Queen's College, Belfast. New Edition. Crown 8vo. price 7s. 6d.

A

The OXFORD REFORMERS—John Colet, Erasmus, and Thomas More; being a History of their Fellow-work. By FREDERIC SEEBOHM. Second Edition, enlarged. 8vo. 14s.

LECTURES on the HISTORY of ENGLAND, from the earliest Times to the Death of King Edward II. By WILLIAM LONGMAN. With Maps and Illustrations. 8vo. 15s.

The HISTORY of the LIFE and TIMES of EDWARD the THIRD. By WILLIAM LONGMAN. With 9 Maps, 8 Plates, and 16 Woodcuts. 2 vols. 8vo. 28s.

The OVERTHROW of the GERMANIC CONFEDERATION by PRUSSIA in 1866. By Sir ALEXANDER MALET, Bart. K.C.B. With 5 Maps. 8vo. 18s.

WATERLOO LECTURES; a Study of the Campaign of 1815. By Colonel CHARLES C. CHESNEY, R.E. late Professor of Military Art and History in the Staff College. New Edition. 8vo. with Map, 10s. 6d.

HISTORY of the REFORMATION in EUROPE in the Time of Calvin. By J. H. MERLE D'AUBIGNÉ, D.D. VOLS. I. and II. 8vo. 28s. VOL. III. 12s. VOL. IV. 16s. VOL. V. price 16s.

ROYAL and REPUBLICAN FRANCE. A Series of Essays reprinted from the Edinburgh, Quarterly, and British and Foreign Reviews. By HENRY REEVE, C.B. D.C.L. 2 vols. 8vo. price 21s.

CHAPTERS from FRENCH HISTORY; St. Louis, Joan of Arc, Henri IV. with Sketches of the Intermediate Periods. By J. H. GURNEY, M.A. New Edition. Fcp. 8vo. 6s. 6d.

MEMOIR of POPE SIXTUS the FIFTH. By Baron HUBNER. Translated from the Original in French, with the Author's sanction, by HUBERT E. H. JERNINGHAM. 2 vols. 8vo. price 24s.   [Nearly ready.

IGNATIUS LOYOLA and the EARLY JESUITS. By STEWART ROSE. New Edition, revised. 8vo. with Portrait, price 16s.

The HISTORY of GREECE. By C. THIRLWALL, D.D. Lord Bishop of St. David's. 8 vols. fcp. 8vo. price 28s.;

GREEK HISTORY from Themistocles to Alexander, in a Series of Lives from Plutarch. Revised and arranged by A. H. CLOUGH. New Edition. Fcp. with 44 Woodcuts, 6s.

CRITICAL HISTORY of the LANGUAGE and LITERATURE of Ancient Greece. By WILLIAM MURE, of Caldwell. 5 vols. 8vo. £3 9s.

The TALE of the GREAT PERSIAN WAR, from the Histories of Herodotus. By GEORGE W. COX, M.A. New Edition. Fcp. 3s. 6d.

HISTORY of the LITERATURE of ANCIENT GREECE. By Professor K. O. MÜLLER. Translated by the Right Hon. Sir GEORGE CORNEWALL LEWIS, Bart. and by J. W. DONALDSON, D.D. 3 vols. 8vo. 21s.

HISTORY of the CITY of ROME from its Foundation to the Sixteenth Century of the Christian Era. By THOMAS H. DYER, LL.D. 8vo. with 2 Maps, 15s.

The HISTORY of ROME. By WILLIAM IHNE. English Edition, translated and revised by the Author. VOLS. I. and II. 8vo. price 30s.

HISTORY of the ROMANS under the EMPIRE. By the Very Rev. C. MERIVALE, D.C.L. Dean of Ely. 8 vols. post 8vo. 48s.

The **FALL** of the **ROMAN REPUBLIC**; a Short History of the **Last** Century of the Commonwealth. By the same Author. 12mo. 7s. 6d.

THREE CENTURIES of **MODERN HISTORY.** By CHARLES DUKE YONGE, B.A. Regius Professor of Modern History and English Literature in Queen's College, Belfast. Crown 8vo. price 7s. 6d.

A STUDENT'S MANUAL of the **HISTORY** of **INDIA**, from the Earliest Period to the Present. By Colonel MEADOWS TAYLOR, M.R.A.S. M.R.I.A. Crown 8vo. with Maps, 7s. 6d.

The **HISTORY** of **INDIA**, from the Earliest Period to the close of Lord Dalhousie's Administration. By JOHN CLARK MARSHMAN. 3 vols. crown 8vo. 22s. 6d.

INDIAN POLITY: a View of the System of Administration in India. By Lieutenant-Colonel GEORGE CHESNEY, Fellow of the University of Calcutta. New Edition, revised; with Map. 8vo. price 21s.

RECREATIONS of an **INDIAN OFFICIAL.** By Lieutenant-Colonel MALLESON, Bengal Staff Corps; Guardian to His Highness the Maharaja of Mysore. Crown 8vo. price 12s. 6d.

HOME POLITICS; being a consideration of the Causes of the Growth of Trade in relation to Labour, Pauperism, and Emigration. By DANIEL GRANT. 8vo. 7s.

REALITIES of **IRISH LIFE.** By W. STEUART TRENCH, Land Agent in Ireland to the Marquess of Lansdowne, the Marquess of Bath, and Lord Digby. Fifth Edition. Crown 8vo. price 6s.

The **STUDENT'S MANUAL** of the **HISTORY** of **IRELAND.** By MARY F. CUSACK, Author of 'The Illustrated History of Ireland, from the Earliest Period to the Year of Catholic Emancipation.' Crown 8vo. price 6s.

CRITICAL and **HISTORICAL ESSAYS** contributed to the *Edinburgh Review.* By the Right Hon. LORD MACAULAY.

CABINET EDITION, 4 vols. post 8vo. 24s. | LIBRARY EDITION, 3 vols. 8vo. 36s. PEOPLE'S EDITION, 2 vols. crown 8vo. 8s. | STUDENT'S EDITION, 1 vol. cr. 8vo. 6s.

SAINT-SIMON and **SAINT-SIMONISM**; a chapter in the History of Socialism in France. By ARTHUR J. BOOTH, M.A. Crown 8vo. price 7s. 6d.

HISTORY of **EUROPEAN MORALS**, from Augustus to Charlemagne. By W. E. H. LECKY, M.A. Second Edition. 2 vols. 8vo. price 28s.

HISTORY of the **RISE** and **INFLUENCE** of the **SPIRIT** of RATIONALISM in EUROPE. By W. E. H. LECKY, M.A. Cabinet Edition, being the Fourth. 2 vols. crown 8vo. price 16s.

GOD in **HISTORY**; or, the Progress of Man's Faith in the Moral Order of the World. By Baron BUNSEN. Translated by SUSANNA WINKWORTH; with a Preface by Dean STANLEY. 3 vols. 8vo. price 42s.

ESSAYS on **HISTORICAL TRUTH.** By ANDREW BISSET. 8vo. 14s.

The **HISTORY** of **PHILOSOPHY**, from Thales to Comte. By GEORGE HENRY LEWES. Fourth Edition. 2 vols. 8vo. 32s.

An **HISTORICAL VIEW** of **LITERATURE** and **ART** in **GREAT BRITAIN** from the Accession of the House of Hanover to the Reign of Queen Victoria. By J. MURRAY GRAHAM, M.A. 8vo. price 14s.

The **MYTHOLOGY** of the **ARYAN NATIONS.** By GEORGE W. Cox, M.A. late Scholar of Trinity College, Oxford, Joint-Editor, with the late Professor Brande, of the Fourth Edition of 'The Dictionary of Science Literature, and Art,' Author of 'Tales of Ancient Greece' &c. 2 vols. 8vo. 28s.

A 2

HISTORY of CIVILISATION in England and France, Spain and 'Scotland. By HENRY THOMAS BUCKLE. !New Edition of the entire Work, with a complete INDEX. 3 vols. crown 8vo. 24s.

HISTORY of the CHRISTIAN CHURCH, from the Ascension of Christ to the Conversion of Constantine. By E. BURTON, D.D. late Prof. of Divinity in the Univ. of Oxford. New Edition. Fcp. 3s. 6d.

SKETCH of the HISTORY of the CHURCH of ENGLAND to the Revolution of 1688. By the Right Rev. T. V. SHORT, D.D. Lord Bishop of St. Asaph. Eighth Edition. Crown 8vo. 7s. 6d.

HISTORY of the EARLY CHURCH, from the First Preaching of the Gospel to the Council of Nicæa. A.D. 325. By ELIZABETH M. SEWELL, Author of 'Amy Herbert.' New Edition, with Questions. Fcp. 4s. 6d.

The ENGLISH REFORMATION. By F. C. MASSINGBERD, M.A. Chancellor of Lincoln and Rector of South Ormsby. Fourth Edition, revised. Fcp. 8vo. 7s. 6d.

MAUNDER'S HISTORICAL TREASURY; comprising a General Introductory Outline of Universal History, and a series of Separate Histories. Latest Edition, revised and brought down to the Present Time by the Rev. GEORGE WILLIAM COX, M.A. Fcp. 6s. cloth, or 9s. 6d. calf.

HISTORICAL and CHRONOLOGICAL ENCYCLOPÆDIA; comprising Chronological Notices of all the Great Events of Universal History: Treaties, Alliances, Wars, Battles, &c.; Incidents in the Lives of Eminent Men and their Works, Scientific and Geographical Discoveries, Mechanical Inventions, and Social, Domestic, and Economical Improvements. By the late B. B. WOODWARD, B.A. and W. L. R. CATES. 1 vol. 8vo. [*Nearly ready.*

Biographical Works.

AUTOBIOGRAPHY of JOHN MILTON; or, Milton's Life in his own Words. By the Rev. JAMES J. G. GRAHAM, M.A. Crown 8vo. price 5s.

A MEMOIR of DANIEL MACLISE, R.A. By W. JUSTIN O'DRISCOLL, M.R.I.A. Barrister-at-Law. With Portrait and Woodcuts. Post 8vo. price 7s. 6d.

MEMOIRS of the MARQUIS of POMBAL; with Extracts from his Writings and from Despatches in the State Papers Office. By the CONDE DA CARNOTA. New Edition. 8vo. price 7s.

LORD GEORGE BENTINCK; a Political Biography. By the Right Hon. BENJAMIN DISRAELI, M.P. Eighth Edition, revised, with a New Preface. Crown 8vo. price 6s.

REMINISCENCES of FIFTY YEARS. By MARK BOYD. Post 8vo. price 10s. 6d.

The LIFE of ISAMBARD KINGDOM BRUNEL, Civil Engineer. By ISAMBARD BRUNEL, B.C.L. of Lincoln's Inn; Chancellor of the Diocese of Ely. With Portrait, Plates, and Woodcuts. 8vo. 21s.

The ROYAL INSTITUTION; its Founder and its First Professors. By Dr. BENCE JONES, Honorary Secretary. Post 8vo. price 12s. 6d.

The LIFE and LETTERS of FARADAY. By Dr. BENCE JONES, Secretary of the Royal Institution. Second Edition, thoroughly revised. 2 vols. 8vo. with Portrait, and Eight Engravings on Wood, price 28s.

FARADAY as a DISCOVERER. By JOHN TYNDALL, LL.D. F.R.S. Professor of Natural Philosophy in the Royal Institution. New and Cheaper Edition, with Two Portraits. Fcp. 8vo. 3s. 6d.

RECOLLECTIONS of PAST LIFE. By Sir HENRY HOLLAND, Bart. M.D. F.R.S. &c. Physician-in-Ordinary to the Queen. Second Edition. Post 8vo. price 10s. 6d.

A GROUP of ENGLISHMEN (1795 to 1815); Records of the Younger Wedgwoods and their Friends, embracing the History of the Discovery of Photography. By ELIZA METEYARD. 8vo. price 16s.

The LIFE and LETTERS of the Rev. SYDNEY SMITH. Edited by his Daughter, Lady HOLLAND, and Mrs. AUSTIN. New Edition, complete in One Volume. Crown 8vo. price 6s.

SOME MEMORIALS of R. D. HAMPDEN, Bishop of Hereford. Edited by his Daughter, HENRIETTA HAMPDEN. With Portrait. 8vo. price 12s.

The LIFE and TRAVELS of GEORGE WHITEFIELD, M.A. By JAMES PATERSON GLEDSTONE. 8vo. price 14s.

LEADERS of PUBLIC OPINION in IRELAND; Swift, Flood, Grattan, O'Connell. By W. E. H. LECKY, M.A. New Edition, revised and enlarged. Crown 8vo. price 7s. 6d.

DICTIONARY of GENERAL BIOGRAPHY; containing Concise Memoirs and Notices of the most Eminent Persons of all Countries, from the Earliest Ages to the Present Time. Edited by W. L. R. CATES. 8vo. 21s.

LIVES of the QUEENS of ENGLAND. By AGNES STRICKLAND. Library Edition, newly revised; with Portraits of every Queen, Autographs, and Vignettes. 8 vols. post 8vo. 7s. 6d. each.

LIFE of the DUKE of WELLINGTON. By the Rev. G. R. GLEIG, M.A. Popular Edition, carefully revised; with copious Additions. Crown 8vo. with Portrait, 5s.

HISTORY of MY RELIGIOUS OPINIONS. By J. H. NEWMAN, D.D. Being the Substance of Apologia pro Vitâ Suâ. Post 8vo. 6s.

The PONTIFICATE of PIUS the NINTH; being the Third Edition of 'Rome and its Ruler,' continued to the latest moment and greatly enlarged. By J. F. MAGUIRE, M.P. Post 8vo. with Portrait, 12s. 6d.

FATHER MATHEW: a Biography. By JOHN FRANCIS MAGUIRE, M.P. for Cork. Popular Edition, with Portrait. Crown 8vo. 3s. 6d.

FELIX MENDELSSOHN'S LETTERS from *Italy and Switzerland*, and *Letters from* 1833 *to* 1847, translated by Lady WALLACE. New Edition, with Portrait. 2 vols. crown 8vo. 5s. each.

MEMOIRS of SIR HENRY HAVELOCK, K.C.B. By JOHN CLARK MARSHMAN. Cabinet Edition, with Portrait. Crown 8vo. price 3s. 6d.

VICISSITUDES of FAMILIES. By Sir J. BERNARD BURKE, C.B. Ulster King of Arms. New Edition, remodelled and enlarged. 2 vols. crown 8vo. 21s.

ESSAYS in ECCLESIASTICAL BIOGRAPHY. By the Right Hon. Sir J. STEPHEN, LL.D. Cabinet Edition, being the Fifth. Crown 8vo. 7s. 6d.

MAUNDER'S BIOGRAPHICAL TREASURY. Thirteenth Edition, reconstructed, thoroughly revised, and in great part rewritten; with about 1,000 additional Memoirs and Notices, by W. L. R. CATES. Fcp. 6s.

LETTERS and LIFE of FRANCIS BACON, including all his Occasional Works. Collected and edited, with a Commentary, by J. SPEDDING, Trin. Coll. Cantab. VOLS. I. and II. 8vo. 24s. VOLS. III. and IV. 24s. VOL. V. price 12s.

Criticism, Philosophy, Polity, &c.

The INSTITUTES of JUSTINIAN; with English Introduction, Translation, and Notes. By T. C. SANDARS, M.A. Barrister, late Fellow of Oriel Coll. Oxon. New Edition. 8vo. 15s.

SOCRATES and the SOCRATIC SCHOOLS. Translated from the German of Dr. E. ZELLER, with the Author's approval, by the Rev. OSWALD J. REICHEL, B.C.L. and M.A. Crown 8vo. 8s. 6d.

The STOICS, EPICUREANS, and SCEPTICS. Translated from the German of Dr. E. ZELLER, with the Author's approval, by OSWALD J. REICHEL, B.C.L. and M.A. Crown 8vo. price 14s.

The ETHICS of ARISTOTLE, illustrated with Essays and Notes. By Sir A. GRANT, Bart. M.A. LL.D. Second Edition, revised and completed. 2 vols. 8vo. price 28s.

The NICOMACHEAN ETHICS of ARISTOTLE newly translated into English. By R. WILLIAMS, B.A. Fellow and late Lecturer of Merton College, and sometime Student of Christ Church, Oxford. 8vo. 12s.

ELEMENTS of LOGIC. By R. WHATELY, D.D. late Archbishop of Dublin. New Edition. 8vo. 10s. 6d. crown 8vo. 4s. 6d.

Elements of Rhetoric. By the same Author. New Edition. 8vo. 10s. 6d. crown 8vo. 4s. 6d.

English Synonymes. By E. JANE WHATELY. Edited by Archbishop WHATELY. 5th Edition. Fcp. 3s.

BACON'S ESSAYS with ANNOTATIONS. By R. WHATELY, D.D. late Archbishop of Dublin. Sixth Edition. 8vo. 10s. 6d.

LORD BACON'S WORKS, collected and edited by J. SPEDDING, M.A. R. L. ELLIS, M.A. and D. D. HEATH. New and Cheaper Edition. 7 vols. 8vo. price £3 13s. 6d.

The SUBJECTION of WOMEN. By JOHN STUART MILL. New Edition. Post 8vo. 5s.

On REPRESENTATIVE GOVERNMENT. By JOHN STUART MILL. Third Edition. 8vo. 9s. Crown 8vo. 2s.

On LIBERTY. By JOHN STUART MILL. Fourth Edition. Post 8vo. 7s. 6d. Crown 8vo. 1s. 4d.

PRINCIPLES of POLITICAL ECONOMY. By the same Author. Seventh Edition. 2 vols. 8vo. 30s. Or in 1 vol. crown 8vo. 5s.

A SYSTEM of LOGIC, RATIOCINATIVE and INDUCTIVE. By the same Author. Seventh Edition. Two vols. 8vo. 25s.

UTILITARIANISM. By JOHN STUART MILL. Fourth Edition. 8vo. 5s.

DISSERTATIONS and DISCUSSIONS, POLITICAL, PHILOSOPHICAL, and HISTORICAL. By JOHN STUART MILL. Second Edition, revised. 3 vols. 8vo. 36s.

EXAMINATION of Sir W. HAMILTON'S PHILOSOPHY, and of the Principal Philosophical Questions discussed in his Writings. By JOHN STUART MILL. Third Edition. 8vo. 16s.

An OUTLINE of the NECESSARY LAWS of THOUGHT: a Treatise on Pure and Applied Logic. By the Most Rev. W. THOMSON, Lord Archbishop of York, D.D. F.R.S. Ninth Thousand. Crown 8vo. 5s. 6d.

The ELEMENTS of POLITICAL ECONOMY. By HENRY DUNNING MACLEOD, M.A. Barrister-at-Law. 8vo. 16s.

A Dictionary of Political Economy; Biographical, Bibliographical, Historical, and Practical. By the same Author. VOL. I. royal 8vo. 30s.

A COLONIST on the COLONIAL QUESTION. By JOHN MATHEWS, of Toronto, Canada. Post 8vo. price 6s.

The ELECTION of REPRESENTATIVES, Parliamentary and Municipal; a Treatise. By THOMAS HARE, Barrister-at-Law. Third Edition, with Additions. Crown 8vo. 6s.

SPEECHES of the RIGHT HON. LORD MACAULAY, corrected by Himself. People's Edition, crown 8vo. 3s. 6d.

Lord Macaulay's Speeches on Parliamentary Reform in 1831 and 1832. 16mo. 1s.

A DICTIONARY of the ENGLISH LANGUAGE. By R. G. LATHAM, M.A. M.D. F.R.S. Founded on the Dictionary of Dr. SAMUEL JOHNSON, as edited by the Rev. H. J. TODD, with numerous Emendations and Additions. In Four Volumes, 4to. price £7.

THESAURUS of ENGLISH WORDS and PHRASES, classified and arranged so as to facilitate the Expression of Ideas, and assist in Literary Composition. By P. M. ROGET, M.D. New Edition. Crown 8vo. 10s. 6d.

LECTURES on the SCIENCE of LANGUAGE. By F. MAX MÜLLER, M.A. &c. Foreign Member of the French Institute. Sixth Edition. 2 vols. crown 8vo. price 16s.

CHAPTERS on LANGUAGE. By FREDERIC W. FARRAR, F.R.S. Head Master of Marlborough College. Crown 8vo. 8s. 6d.

MANUAL of ENGLISH LITERATURE, Historical and Critical. By THOMAS ARNOLD, M.A. Second Edition. Crown 8vo. price 7s. 6d.

THREE CENTURIES of ENGLISH LITERATURE. By CHARLES DUKE YONGE, Regius Professor of Modern History and English Literature in Queen's College, Belfast. Crown 8vo. price 7s. 6d.

SOUTHEY'S DOCTOR, complete in One Volume. Edited by the Rev. J. W. WARTER, B.D. Square crown 8vo. 12s. 6d.

HISTORICAL and CRITICAL COMMENTARY on the OLD TESTAMENT; with a New Translation. By M. M. KALISCH, Ph.D. VOL. I. *Genesis*, 8vo. 18s. or adapted for the General Reader, 12s. VOL. II. *Exodus*, 15s. or adapted for the General Reader, 12s. VOL. III. *Leviticus*. PART I. 15s. or adapted for the General Reader. 8s. VOL. IV. *Leviticus*, PART II. 15s. or adapted for the General Reader, 8s.

A HEBREW GRAMMAR, with EXERCISES. By M. M. KALISCH, Ph.D. PART I. *Outlines with Exercises*, 8vo. 12s. 6d. KEY, 5s. PART II. *Exceptional Forms and Constructions*, 12s. 6d.

A LATIN-ENGLISH DICTIONARY. By JOHN T. WHITE, D.D. Oxon. and J. E. RIDDLE, M.A. Oxon. Third Edition, revised. 2 vols. 4to. pp. 2,128, price 42s. cloth.

White's College Latin-English Dictionary (Intermediate Size), abridged for the use of University Students from the Parent Work (as above). Medium 8vo. pp. 1,048, price 18s. cloth.

White's Junior Student's Complete Latin-English and English-Latin Dictionary. New Edition. Square 12mo. pp. 1,058, price 12s.

Separately { The ENGLISH-LATIN DICTIONARY, price 5s. 6d.
              The LATIN-ENGLISH DICTIONARY, price 7s. 6d.

An ENGLISH-GREEK LEXICON, containing all the Greek Words used by Writers of good authority. By C. D. YONGE, B.A. New Edition. 4to. 21s.

Mr. YONGE'S NEW LEXICON, English and Greek, abridged from his larger work (as above). Revised Edition. Square 12mo. 8s. 6d.

A GREEK-ENGLISH LEXICON. Compiled by H. G. LIDDELL, D.D. Dean of Christ Church, and R. SCOTT, D.D. Dean of Rochester. Sixth Edition. Crown 4to. price 36s.

A Lexicon, Greek and English, abridged from LIDDELL and SCOTT's *Greek-English Lexicon*. Fourteenth Edition. Square 12mo. 7s. 6d.

A SANSKRIT-ENGLISH DICTIONARY, the Sanskrit words printed both in the original Devanagari and in Roman Letters. Compiled by T. BENFEY, Prof. in the Univ. of Göttingen. 8vo. 52s. 6d.

WALKER'S PRONOUNCING DICTIONARY of the ENGLISH LAN-GUAGE. Thoroughly revised Editions, by B. H. SMART. 8vo. 12s. 16mo. 6s.

A PRACTICAL DICTIONARY of the FRENCH and ENGLISH LAN-GUAGES. By L. CONTANSEAU. Fourteenth Edition. Post 8vo. 10s. 6d.

Contanseau's Pocket Dictionary, French and English, abridged from the above by the Author. New Edition, revised. Square 18mo. 3s. 6d.

NEW PRACTICAL DICTIONARY of the GERMAN LANGUAGE; German-English and English-German. By the Rev. W. L. BLACKLEY, M.A. and Dr. CARL MARTIN FRIEDLÄNDER. Post 8vo. 7s. 6d.

The MASTERY of LANGUAGES; or, the Art of Speaking Foreign Tongues Idiomatically. By THOMAS PRENDERGAST, late of the Civil Service at Madras. Second Edition. 8vo. 6s,

---

Miscellaneous Works and Popular Metaphysics.

The ESSAYS and CONTRIBUTIONS of A. K. H. B., Author of 'The Recreations of a Country Parson.' Uniform Editions:—

Recreations of a Country Parson. By A. K. H. B. FIRST and SECOND SERIES, crown 8vo. 3s. 6d. each.

The COMMON-PLACE PHILOSOPHER in TOWN and COUNTRY. By A. K. H. B. Crown 8vo. price 3s. 6d.

Leisure Hours in Town; Essays Consolatory, Æsthetical, Moral, Social, and Domestic. By A. K. H. B. Crown 8vo. 3s. 6d.

The AUTUMN HOLIDAYS of a COUNTRY PARSON; Essays contributed to *Fraser's Magazine* and to *Good Words*. By A.K.H.B. Crown 8vo. 3s. 6d.

The Graver Thoughts of a Country Parson. By A. K. H. B. FIRST and SECOND SERIES, crown 8vo. 3s. 6d. each.

Critical Essays of a Country Parson, selected from Essays contributed to *Fraser's Magazine*. By A.K.H.B. Crown 8vo. 3s. 6d.

Sunday Afternoons at the Parish Church of a Scottish University City. By A. K. H. B. Crown 8vo. 3s. 6d.

Lessons of Middle Age; with some Account of various Cities and Men. By A. K. H. B. Crown 8vo. 3s. 6d.

Counsel and Comfort spoken from a City Pulpit. By A. K. H. B. Crown 8vo. price 3s. 6d.

Changed Aspects of Unchanged Truths; Memorials of St. Andrews Sundays. By A. K. H.B. Crown 8vo. 3s. 6d.

Present-day Thoughts; Memorials of St. Andrews Sundays. By A. K. H. B. Crown 8vo. 3s. 6d.

SHORT STUDIES on GREAT SUBJECTS. By JAMES ANTHONY FROUDE, M.A., late Fellow of Exeter Coll. Oxford. 2 vols. 8vo. price 24s.

LORD MACAULAY'S MISCELLANEOUS WRITINGS:—

LIBRARY EDITION. 2 vols. 8vo. Portrait, 21s.
PEOPLE'S EDITION. 1 vol. crown 8vo. 4s. 6d.

LORD MACAULAY'S MISCELLANEOUS WRITINGS and SPEECHES. STUDENT'S EDITION, in crown 8vo. price 6s.

The REV. SYDNEY SMITH'S MISCELLANEOUS WORKS; including his Contributions to the *Edinburgh Review*. Crown 8vo. 6s.

The Wit and Wisdom of the Rev. Sydney Smith; a Selection of the most memorable Passages in his Writings and Conversation. 16mo. 3s. 6d.

The ECLIPSE of FAITH; or, a Visit to a Religious Sceptic. By HENRY ROGERS. Twelfth Edition. Fcp. 5s.

Defence of the Eclipse of Faith, by its Author; a rejoinder to Dr. Newman's *Reply*. Third Edition. Fcp. 3s. 6d.

Selections from the Correspondence of R. E. H. Greyson. By the same Author. Third Edition. Crown 8vo. 7s. 6d.

FAMILIES of SPEECH, Four Lectures delivered at the Royal Institution of Great Britain. By the Rev. F. W. FARRAR, M.A. F.R.S. Head Master of Marlborough College. Post 8vo. with Two Maps, 5s. 6d.

CHIPS from a GERMAN WORKSHOP; being Essays on the Science of Religion, and on Mythology, Traditions, and Customs. By F. MAX MÜLLER, M.A. &c. Foreign Member of the French Institute. 3 vols. 8vo. £2.

UEBERWEG'S SYSTEM of LOGIC and HISTORY of LOGICAL DOCTRINES. Translated, with Notes and Appendices, by T. M. LINDSAY, M.A. F.R.S.E. Examiner in Philosophy to the University of Edinburgh. 8vo. price 16s.

ANALYSIS of the PHENOMENA of the HUMAN MIND. By JAMES MILL. A New Edition, with Notes, Illustrative and Critical, by ALEXANDER BAIN, ANDREW FINDLATER, and GEORGE GROTE. Edited, with additional Notes, by JOHN STUART MILL. 2 vols. 8vo. price 28s.

An **INTRODUCTION** to **MENTAL PHILOSOPHY**, on the Inductive Method. By J. D. MORELL, M.A. LL.D. 8vo. 12s.

ELEMENTS of **PSYCHOLOGY**, containing the Analysis of the Intellectual Powers. By the same Author. Post 8vo. 7s. 6d.

The **SECRET** of **HEGEL**: being the Hegelian System in Origin, Principle, Form, and Matter. By J. H. STIRLING. 2 vols. 8vo. 28s.

SIR WILLIAM HAMILTON; being the Philosophy of Perception: an Analysis. By J. H. STIRLING. 8vo. 5s.

The **SENSES** and the **INTELLECT**. By ALEXANDER BAIN, M.D. Professor of Logic in the University of Aberdeen. Third Edition. 8vo. 15s.

MENTAL and **MORAL SCIENCE**: a Compendium of Psychology and Ethics. By the same Author. Second Edition. Crown 8vo. 10s. 6d.

LOGIC, DEDUCTIVE and **INDUCTIVE**. By the same Author. In TWO PARTS, crown 8vo. 10s. 6d. Each Part may be had separately:— PART I. *Deduction*, 4s. PART II. *Induction*, 6s. 6d.

TIME and **SPACE**; a Metaphysical Essay. By SHADWORTH H. HODGSON. (This work covers the whole ground of Speculative Philosophy.) 8vo. price 16s.

The Theory of Practice; an Ethical Inquiry. By the same Author. (This work, in conjunction with the foregoing, completes a system of Philosophy.) 2 vols. 8vo. price 24s.

The **PHILOSOPHY** of **NECESSITY**; or, Natural Law as applicable to Mental, Moral, and Social Science. By CHARLES BRAY. Second Edition. 8vo. 9s.

A Manual of Anthropology, or Science of Man, based on Modern Research. By the same Author. Crown 8vo. price 6s.

On Force, its Mental and Moral Correlates. By the same Author. 8vo. 5s.

The **DISCOVERY** of a **NEW WORLD** of **BEING**. By GEORGE THOMSON. Post 8vo. price 6s.

A **TREATISE** on **HUMAN NATURE**; being an Attempt to Introduce the Experimental Method of Reasoning into Moral Subjects. By DAVID HUME. Edited, with Notes, &c. by T. H. GREEN, Fellow, and T. H. GROSE, late Scholar, of Balliol College, Oxford.   [*In the press.*

ESSAYS MORAL, POLITICAL, and **LITERARY**. By DAVID HUME. By the same Editors.   [*In the press.*

Astronomy, Meteorology, Popular Geography, &c.

OUTLINES of **ASTRONOMY**. By Sir J. F. W. HERSCHEL, Bart. M.A. Eleventh Edition, with 9 Plates and numerous Diagrams. Square crown 8vo. price 12s.

ESSAYS on **ASTRONOMY**. By RICHARD A. PROCTOR, B.A. Hon. Sec. R.A.S. (Dedicated, by permission, to the Astronomer Royal.) 8vo. with 10 Plates and 20 Wood Engravings, price 12s.

The SUN; RULER, LIGHT, FIRE, and LIFE of the PLANETARY SYSTEM. By RICHARD A. PROCTOR, B.A. F.R.A.S. With 10 Plates (7 coloured) and 107 Figures on Wood. Crown 8vo. 14s.

OTHER WORLDS THAN OURS; the Plurality of Worlds Studied under the Light of Recent Scientific Researches. By the same Author. Second Edition, with 14 Illustrations. Crown 8vo. 10s. 6d.

SATURN and its SYSTEM. By the same Author. 8vo. with 14 Plates, 14s.

SCHELLEN'S SPECTRUM ANALYSIS, in its application to Terrestrial Substances and the Physical Constitution of the Heavenly Bodies. Translated by JANE and C. LASSELL; edited, with Notes, by W. HUGGINS, LL.D. F.R.S. With 13 Plates (6 coloured) and 223 Woodcuts. 8vo. price 28s.

A NEW STAR ATLAS, for the Library, the School, and the Observatory, in Twelve Circular Maps (with Two Index Plates). Intended as a Companion to 'Webb's Celestial Objects for Common Telescopes.' With a Letterpress Introduction on the Study of the Stars, illustrated by 9 Diagrams. By RICHARD A. PROCTOR, B.A. Hon. Sec. R.A.S. Crown 8vo. 5s.

CELESTIAL OBJECTS for COMMON TELESCOPES. By the Rev. T. W. WEBB, M.A. F.R.A.S. Third Edition, revised, with a large Map of the Moon, and several Woodcuts. 16mo. 7s. 6d.

NAVIGATION and NAUTICAL ASTRONOMY (Practical, Theoretical, Scientific) for the use of Students and Practical Men. By J. MERRIFIELD, F.R.A.S and H. EVERS. 8vo. 14s.

DOVE'S LAW of STORMS, considered in connexion with the Ordinary Movements of the Atmosphere. Translated by R. H. SCOTT, M.A. T.C.D. 8vo. 10s. 6d.

A GENERAL DICTIONARY of GEOGRAPHY, Descriptive, Physical, Statistical, and Historical : forming a complete Gazetteer of the World. By A. KEITH JOHNSTON, LL.D. F.R.G.S. Revised Edition. 8vo. 31s. 6d.

A MANUAL of GEOGRAPHY, Physical, Industrial, and Political. By W. HUGHES, F.R.G.S. With 6 Maps. Fcp. 7s. 6d.

MAUNDER'S TREASURY of GEOGRAPHY, Physical, Historical, Descriptive, and Political. Edited by W. HUGHES, F.R.G.S. Revised Edition, with 7 Maps and 16 Plates. Fcp. 6s. cloth, or 9s. 6d. bound in calf.

The PUBLIC SCHOOLS ATLAS of MODERN GEOGRAPHY. In 31 Maps, exhibiting clearly the more important Physical Features of the Countries delineated, and Noting all the Chief Places of Historical, Commercial, or Social Interest. Edited, with an Introduction, by the Rev. G. BUTLER, M.A. Imp. 4to. price 3s. 6d. sewed, or 5s. cloth.

Natural History and Popular Science.

TEXT-BOOKS of SCIENCE, MECHANICAL and PHYSICAL. Edited by T. M. GOODEVE, M.A. The following may now be had, price 3s. 6d. each :—
    1.　GOODEVE'S Mechanism.
    2.　BLOXAM'S Metals.
    3.　MILLER'S Inorganic Chemistry.
    4.　GRIFFIN'S Algebra and Trigonometry.
    5.　WATSON'S Plane and Solid Geometry.
    6.　MAXWELL'S Theory of Heat.
    7.　MERRIFIELD'S Technical Arithmetic and Mensuration.

ELEMENTARY TREATISE on PHYSICS, Experimental and Applied. Translated and edited from GANOT's *Eléments de Physique* (with the Author's sanction) by E. ATKINSON, Ph.D. F.C.S. New Edition, revised and enlarged; with a Coloured Plate and 726 Woodcuts. Post 8vo. 15s.

NATURAL PHILOSOPHY for GENERAL READERS and YOUNG PERSONS; being a Course of Physics divested of Mathematical Formulæ, expressed in the language of daily life, and illustrated with Explanatory Figures, familiarly elucidating the Principles and Facts. Translated and edited from GANOT's *Cours de Physique*, with the Author's sanction, by E. ATKINSON, Ph.D. F.C.S. Crown 8vo. with Woodcuts, price 7s. 6d.

SOUND: a Course of Eight Lectures delivered at the Royal Institution of Great Britain. By JOHN TYNDALL, LL.D. F.R.S. New Edition, crown 8vo. with Portrait of *M. Chladni* and 169 Woodcuts, price 9s.

HEAT a MODE of MOTION. By Professor JOHN TYNDALL, LL.D. F.R.S. Fourth Edition. Crown 8vo. with Woodcuts, 10s. 6d.

RESEARCHES in MOLECULAR PHYSICS by MEANS of RADIANT HEAT; a Series of Memoirs collected from the Philosophical Transactions. By JOHN TYNDALL, LL.D. F.R.S. 1 vol. 8vo. [*In the press.*

RESEARCHES on DIAMAGNETISM and MAGNE-CRYSTALLIC ACTION; including the Question of Diamagnetic Polarity. By the same Author. With 6 Plates and many Woodcuts. 8vo. price 14s.

NOTES of a COURSE of SEVEN LECTURES on ELECTRICAL PHENOMENA and THEORIES, delivered at the Royal Institution, A.D. 1870. By Professor TYNDALL. Crown 8vo. 1s. sewed, or 1s. 6d. cloth.

NOTES of a COURSE of NINE LECTURES on LIGHT delivered at the Royal Institution, A.D. 1869. By the same Author. Crown 8vo. price 1s. sewed, or 1s. 6d. cloth.

FRAGMENTS of SCIENCE. By JOHN TYNDALL, LL.D. F.R.S. Third Edition. 8vo. price 14s.

LIGHT SCIENCE for LEISURE HOURS; a Series of Familiar Essays on Scientific Subjects, Natural Phenomena, &c. By R. A. PROCTOR, B.A. F.R.A.S. Crown 8vo. price 7s. 6d.

LIGHT: Its Influence on Life and Health. By FORBES WINSLOW, M.D. D.C.L. Oxon. (Hon.). Fcp. 8vo. 6s.

A TREATISE on ELECTRICITY, in Theory and Practice. By A. DE LA RIVE, Prof. in the Academy of Geneva. Translated by C. V. WALKER F.R.S. 3 vols. 8vo. with Woodcuts, £3 13s.

The CORRELATION of PHYSICAL FORCES. By W. R. GROVE, Q.C. V.P.R.S. Fifth Edition, revised, and followed by a Discourse on Continuity. 8vo. 10s. 6d. The *Discourse on Continuity*, separately, 2s. 6d.

VAN DER HOEVEN'S HANDBOOK of ZOOLOGY. Translated from the Second Dutch Edition by the Rev. W. CLARK, M.D. F.R.S. 2 vols. 8vo. with 24 Plates of Figures, 60s.

Professor OWEN'S LECTURES on the COMPARATIVE ANATOMY and Physiology of the Invertebrate Animals. Second Edition, with 235 Woodcuts. 8vo. 21s.

The COMPARATIVE ANATOMY and PHYSIOLOGY of the VERTE-brate Animals. By RICHARD OWEN, F.R.S. D.C.L. With 1,472 Woodcuts. 3 vols. 8vo. £3 13s. 6d.

The **ORIGIN of CIVILISATION** and the **PRIMITIVE CONDITION** of MAN; Mental and Social Condition of Savages. By Sir JOHN LUBBOCK, Bart. M.P. F.R.S. Second Edition, with 25 Woodcuts. 8vo. price 16s.

The **PRIMITIVE INHABITANTS of SCANDINAVIA**: containing a Description of the Implements, Dwellings, Tombs, and Mode of Living of the Savages in the North of Europe during the Stone Age. By SVEN NILSSON. With 16 Plates of Figures and 3 Woodcuts. 8vo. 18s.

BIBLE ANIMALS; being a Description of every Living Creature mentioned in the Scriptures, from the Ape to the Coral. By the Rev. J. G. WOOD, M.A. F.L.S. With about 100 Vignettes on Wood. 8vo. 21s.

HOMES WITHOUT HANDS; a Description of the Habitations of Animals, classed according to their Principle of Construction. By the Rev. J. G. WOOD, M.A. F.L.S. With about 140 Vignettes on Wood. 8vo. 21s.

INSECTS AT HOME; a Popular Account of British Insects, their Structure, Habits, and Transformations. By the Rev. J. G. WOOD, M.A. F.L.S. With upwards of 700 Illustrations engraved on Wood (1 coloured and 21 full size of page). 8vo. price 21s.

STRANGE DWELLINGS; a description of the Habitations of Animals, abridged from 'Homes without Hands.' By the Rev. J. G. WOOD, M.A. F.L.S. With about 60 Woodcut Illustrations. Crown 8vo. price 7s. 6d.

A FAMILIAR HISTORY of BIRDS. By E. STANLEY, D.D. F.R.S. late Lord Bishop of Norwich. Seventh Edition, with Woodcuts. Fcp. 3s. 6d.

The **HARMONIES of NATURE** and **UNITY of CREATION.** By Dr. GEORGE HARTWIG. 8vo. with numerous Illustrations, 18s.

The **SEA** and its **LIVING WONDERS.** By the same Author. Third (English) Edition. 8vo. with many Illustrations, 21s.

The **TROPICAL WORLD.** By Dr. GEO. HARTWIG. With 8 Chromo-xylographs and 172 Woodcuts. 8vo. 21s.

The **SUBTERRANEAN WORLD.** By Dr. GEORGE HARTWIG. With 3 Maps and about 80 Woodcuts, including 8 full size of page. 8vo. price 21s.

The **POLAR WORLD**, a Popular Description of Man and Nature in the Arctic and Antarctic Regions of the Globe. By Dr. GEORGE HARTWIG. With 8 Chromoxylographs, 3 Maps, and 85 Woodcuts. 8vo. 21s.

KIRBY and **SPENCE'S INTRODUCTION** to **ENTOMOLOGY,** or Elements of the Natural History of Insects. 7th Edition. Crown 8vo. 5s.

MAUNDER'S TREASURY of NATURAL HISTORY, or Popular Dictionary of Zoology. Revised and corrected by T. S. COBBOLD, M.D. Fcp. with 900 Woodcuts, 6s. cloth, or 9s. 6d. bound in calf.

The **TREASURY of BOTANY,** or Popular Dictionary of the Vegetable Kingdom; including a Glossary of Botanical Terms. Edited by J. LINDLEY, F.R.S. and T. MOORE, F.L.S. assisted by eminent Contributors. With 274 Woodcuts and 20 Steel Plates. Two Parts, fcp. 12s. cloth, or 19s. calf.

The **ELEMENTS of BOTANY** for **FAMILIES** and **SCHOOLS.** Tenth Edition, revised by THOMAS MOORE, F.L.S. Fcp. with 154 Woodcuts. 2s. 6d.

The **ROSE AMATEUR'S GUIDE.** By THOMAS RIVERS. Ninth Edition. Fcp. 4s.

LOUDON'S ENCYCLOPÆDIA of PLANTS; comprising the Specific Character, Description, Culture, History, &c. of all the Plants found in Great Britain. With upwards of 12,000 Woodcuts. 8vo. 42s.

MAUNDER'S SCIENTIFIC and LITERARY TREASURY. New Edition, thoroughly revised and in great part re-written, with above 1,000 new Articles, by J. Y. JOHNSON, Corr. M.Z.S. Fcp. 6s. cloth, or 9s. 6d. calf.

A DICTIONARY of SCIENCE, LITERATURE, and ART. Fourth Edition, re-edited by W. T. BRANDE (the original Author), and GEORGE W. COX, M.A. assisted by contributors of eminent Scientific and Literary Acquirements. 3 vols. medium 8vo. price 63s. cloth.

Chemistry, Medicine, Surgery, and the Allied Sciences.

A DICTIONARY of CHEMISTRY and the Allied Branches of other Sciences. By HENRY WATTS, F.R.S. assisted by eminent Contributors Complete in 5 vols. medium 8vo. £7 3s.

Supplement; bringing the Record of Chemical Discovery down to the end of the year 1869; including also several Additions to, and Corrections of, former results which have appeared in 1870 and 1871. By HENRY WATTS, B.A. F.R.S. F.C.S. Assisted by eminent Scientific and Practical Chemists, Contributors to the Original Work. 8vo. price 31s. 6d.

ELEMENTS of CHEMISTRY, Theoretical and Practical. By W. ALLEN MILLER, M.D. late Prof. of Chemistry, King's Coll. London. Fourth Edition. 3 vols. 8vo. £3. PART I. CHEMICAL PHYSICS, 15s. PART II. INORGANIC CHEMISTRY, 21s. PART III. ORGANIC CHEMISTRY, 24s.

OUTLINES of CHEMISTRY; or, Brief Notes of Chemical Facts. By WILLIAM ODLING, M.B. F.R.S. Crown 8vo. 7s. 6d.

A Course of Practical Chemistry, for the use of Medical Students. By the same Author. New Edition, with 70 Woodcuts. Crown 8vo. 7s. 6d.

Lectures on Animal Chemistry, delivered at the Royal College of Physicians in 1865. By the same Author. Crown 8vo. 4s. 6d.

SELECT METHODS in CHEMICAL ANALYSIS, chiefly INOR-GANIC. By WILLIAM CROOKES, F.R.S. With 22 Woodcuts. Crown 8vo. price 12s. 6d.

CHEMICAL NOTES for the LECTURE ROOM. By THOMAS WOOD, F.C.S. 2 vols. crown 8vo. I. on Heat &c. price 5s. II. on the Metals, 5s.

The DIAGNOSIS, PATHOLOGY, and TREATMENT of DISEASES of Women; including the Diagnosis of Pregnancy. By GRAILY HEWITT, M.D. Second Edition, enlarged; with 116 Woodcut Illustrations. 8vo. 24s.

On SOME DISORDERS of the NERVOUS SYSTEM in CHILD-HOOD; being the Lumleian Lectures delivered before the Royal College of Physicians in March 1871. By CHARLES WEST, M.D. Crown 8vo. price 5s.

LECTURES on the DISEASES of INFANCY and CHILDHOOD. By CHARLES WEST, M.D. &c. Fifth Edition, revised and enlarged. 8vo. 16s.

A SYSTEM of SURGERY, Theoretical and Practical. In Treatises by Various Authors. Edited by T. HOLMES, M.A. &c. Surgeon and Lecturer on Surgery at St. George's Hospital, and Surgeon-in-Chief to the Metropolitan Police. Second Edition, thoroughly revised, with numerous Illustrations. 5 vols. 8vo. £5 5s.

The SURGICAL TREATMENT of CHILDREN'S DISEASES. By T. HOLMES, M.A. &c. late Surgeon to the Hospital for Sick Children. Second Edition, with 9 Plates and 112 Woodcuts. 8vo. 21s.

LECTURES on the PRINCIPLES and PRACTICE of PHYSIC. By Sir THOMAS WATSON, Bart. M.D. Fifth Edition, thoroughly revised. 2 vols. 8vo. price 36s.

LECTURES on SURGICAL PATHOLOGY. By Sir JAMES PAGET, Bart. F.R.S. Third Edition, revised and re-edited by the Author and Professor W. TURNER, M.B. 8vo. with 131 Woodcuts, 21s.

COOPER'S DICTIONARY of PRACTICAL SURGERY and Encyclopædia of Surgical Science. New Edition, brought down to the present time. By S. A. LANE, Surgeon to St. Mary's Hospital, assisted by various Eminent Surgeons. VOL. II. 8vo. completing the work. [*In the press.*

On CHRONIC BRONCHITIS, especially as connected with GOUT, EMPHYSEMA, and DISEASES of the HEART. By E. HEADLAM GREENHOW, M.D. F.R.C.P. &c. 8vo. 7s. 6d.

The CLIMATE of the SOUTH of FRANCE as SUITED to INVALIDS; with Notices of Mediterranean and other Winter Stations. By C. T. WILLIAMS, M.A. M.D. Oxon. Assistant-Physician to the Hospital for Consumption at Brompton. Second Edition. Crown 8vo. 6s.

REPORTS on the PROGRESS of PRACTICAL and SCIENTIFIC MEDICINE in Different Parts of the World. Edited by HORACE DOBELL, M.D. assisted by numerous and distinguished Coadjutors. Vols. I. and II. 8vo. 18s. each.

PULMONARY CONSUMPTION; its Nature, Varieties, and Treatment : with an Analysis of One Thousand Cases to exemplify its Duration. By C. J. B. WILLIAMS, M.D. F.R.S. and C. T. WILLIAMS, M.A. M.D. Oxon. Post 8vo. price 10s. 6d.

CLINICAL LECTURES on DISEASES of the LIVER, JAUNDICE, and ABDOMINAL DROPSY. By CHARLES MURCHISON, M.D. Post 8vo. with 25 Woodcuts, 10s. 6d.

ANATOMY, DESCRIPTIVE and SURGICAL. By HENRY GRAY, F.R.S. With about 400 Woodcuts from Dissections. Fifth Edition, by T. HOLMES, M.A. Cantab. with a new Introduction by the Editor. Royal 8vo. 28s.

OUTLINES of PHYSIOLOGY, Human and Comparative. By JOHN MARSHALL, F.R.C.S. Surgeon to the University College Hospital. 2 vols. crown 8vo. with 122 Woodcuts, 32s.

PHYSIOLOGICAL ANATOMY and PHYSIOLOGY of MAN. By the late R. B. TODD, M.D. F.R.S. and W. BOWMAN, F.R.S. of King's College. With numerous Illustrations. VOL. II. 8vo. 25s.
VOL. I. New Edition by Dr. LIONEL S. BEALE. F.R.S. in course of publication, with many Illustrations. PARTS I. and II. price 7s. 6d. each.

COPLAND'S DICTIONARY of PRACTICAL MEDICINE, abridged from the larger work and throughout brought down to the present State of Medical Science. 8vo. 36s.

On the **MANUFACTURE** of **BEET-ROOT SUGAR** in **ENGLAND** and IRELAND. By WILLIAM CROOKES, F.R.S. Crown 8vo. with 11 Woodcuts, 8s. 6d.

DR. **PEREIRA'S ELEMENTS** of **MATERIA MEDICA** and **THERA-**PEUTICS, abridged and adapted for the use of Medical and Pharmaceutical Practitioners and Students; and comprising all the Medicines of the British Pharmacopœia, with such others as are frequently ordered in Pre-scriptions or required by the Physician. Edited by Professor BENTLEY, F.L.S. &c. and by Dr. REDWOOD, F.C.S. &c. With 125 Woodcut Illustra-tions. 8vo. price 25s.

The Fine Arts, and Illustrated Editions.

IN FAIRYLAND; Pictures from the Elf-World. By RICHARD DOYLE. With a Poem by W. ALLINGHAM. With Sixteen Plates, containing Thirty-six Designs printed in Colours. Folio, 31s. 6d.

HALF-HOUR LECTURES on the **HISTORY** and **PRACTICE** of the Fine and Ornamental Arts. By WILLIAM B. SCOTT. New Edition, revised by the Author; with 50 Woodcuts. Crown 8vo. 8s. 6d.

ALBERT DURER, HIS LIFE and **WORKS**; including Auto-biographical Papers and Complete Catalogues. By WILLIAM B. SCOTT. With Six Etchings by the Author, and other Illustrations. 8vo. 16s.

The **CHORALE BOOK** for **ENGLAND**: the Hymns translated by Miss C. WINKWORTH; the Tunes arranged by Prof. W. S. BENNETT and OTTO GOLDSCHMIDT. Fcp. 4to. 12s. 6d.

The **NEW TESTAMENT**, illustrated with Wood Engravings after the Early Masters, chiefly of the Italian School. Crown 4to. 63s. cloth, gilt top ; or £5 5s. elegantly bound in morocco.

LYRA GERMANICA; the Christian Year. Translated by CATHERINE WINKWORTH; with 125 Illustrations on Wood drawn by J. LEIGHTON, F.S.A. 4to. 21s.

LYRA GERMANICA; the Christian Life. Translated by CATHERINE WINKWORTH; with about 200 Woodcut Illustrations by J. LEIGHTON, F.S.A. and other Artists. 4to. 21s.

The **LIFE** of **MAN SYMBOLISED** by the **MONTHS** of the **YEAR**. Text selected by R. PIGOT ; Illustrations on Wood from Original Designs by J. LEIGHTON, F.S.A. 4to. 42s.

CATS' and **FARLIE'S MORAL EMBLEMS**; with Aphorisms, Adages, and Proverbs of all Nations. 121 Illustrations on Wood by J. LEIGHTON, F.S.A. Text selected by R. PIGOT. Imperial 8vo. 31s. 6d.

SACRED and **LEGENDARY ART**. By Mrs. JAMESON.

Legends of the Saints and Martyrs. New Edition, with 19 Etchings and 187 Woodcuts. 2 vols. square crown 8vo. 31s. 6d.

Legends of the Monastic Orders. New Edition, with 11 Etchings and 88 Woodcuts. 1 vol. square crown 8vo. 21s.

SACRED and LEGENDARY ART. By Mrs. JAMESON.

Legends of the Madonna. New Edition, with 27 Etchings and 165 Woodcuts. 1 vol. square crown 8vo. 21s.

The History of Our Lord, with that of his Types and Precursors. Completed by Lady EASTLAKE. Revised Edition, with 31 Etchings and 281 Woodcuts. 2 vols. square crown 8vo. 42s.

The Useful Arts, Manufactures, &c.

HISTORY of the GOTHIC REVIVAL; an Attempt to shew how far the taste for Mediæval Architecture was retained in England during the last two centuries, and has been re-developed in the present. By C. L. EASTLAKE, Architect. With 48 Illustrations (36 full size of page). Imperial 8vo. price 31s. 6d.

GWILT'S ENCYCLOPÆDIA of ARCHITECTURE, with above 1,600 Engravings on Wood. Fifth Edition, revised and enlarged by WYATT PAPWORTH. 8vo. 52s. 6d.

A MANUAL of ARCHITECTURE: being a Concise History and Explanation of the principal Styles of European Architecture, Ancient, Mediæval, and Renaissance; with a Glossary of Technical Terms. By THOMAS MITCHELL. Crown 8vo. with 150 Woodcuts, 10s. 6d.

HINTS on HOUSEHOLD TASTE in FURNITURE, UPHOLSTERY, and other Details. By CHARLES L. EASTLAKE, Architect. Second Edition, with about 90 Illustrations. Square crown 8vo. 18s.

PRINCIPLES of MECHANISM, designed for the Use of Students in the Universities, and for Engineering Students generally. By R. WILLIS, M.A. F.R.S. &c. Jacksonian Professor in the University of Cambridge. Second Edition, enlarged; with 374 Woodcuts. 8vo. 18s.

LATHES and TURNING, Simple, Mechanical, and ORNAMENTAL. By W. HENRY NORTHCOTT. With about 240 Illustrations on Steel and Wood. 8vo. 18s.

URE'S DICTIONARY of ARTS, MANUFACTURES, and MINES. Sixth Edition, chiefly rewritten and greatly enlarged by ROBERT HUNT, F.R.S. assisted by numerous Contributors eminent in Science and the Arts, and familiar with Manufactures. With above 2,000 Woodcuts. 3 vols. medium 8vo. price £4 14s. 6d.

HANDBOOK of PRACTICAL TELEGRAPHY. By R. S. CULLEY, Memb. Inst. C.E. Engineer-in-Chief of Telegraphs to the Post Office. Fifth Edition, with 118 Woodcuts and 9 Plates. 8vo. price 14s.

ENCYCLOPÆDIA of CIVIL ENGINEERING, Historical, Theoretical, and Practical. By E. CRESY, C.E. With above 3,000 Woodcuts. 8vo. 42s.

TREATISE on MILLS and MILLWORK. By Sir W. FAIRBAIRN, Bart. F.R.S. New Edition, with 18 Plates and 322 Woodcuts. 2 vols. 8vo. 32s.

USEFUL INFORMATION for ENGINEERS. By the same Author. FIRST, SECOND, and THIRD SERIES, with many Plates and Woodcuts, 3 vols. crown 8vo. 10s. 6d. each.

The APPLICATION of CAST and WROUGHT IRON to Building Purposes. By Sir W. FAIRBAIRN, Bart. F.R.S. Fourth Edition, enlarged; with 6 Plates and 118 Woodcuts. 8vo. price 16s.

B

IRON SHIP BUILDING, its History and Progress, as comprised in a Series of Experimental Researches. By the same Author. With 4 Plates and 130 Woodcuts. 8vo. 18s.

A TREATISE on the STEAM ENGINE, in its various Applications to Mines, Mills, Steam Navigation, Railways and Agriculture. By J. BOURNE, C.E. Eighth Edition; with Portrait, 37 Plates, and 546 Woodcuts. 4to. 42s.

CATECHISM of the STEAM ENGINE, in its various Applications to Mines, Mills, Steam Navigation, Railways, and Agriculture. By the same Author. With 89 Woodcuts. Fcp. 6s.

HANDBOOK of the STEAM ENGINE. By the same Author, forming a KEY to the Catechism of the Steam Engine, with 67 Woodcuts. Fcp. 9s.

BOURNE'S RECENT IMPROVEMENTS in the STEAM ENGINE in its various applications to Mines, Mills, Steam Navigation, Railways, and Agriculture. Being a Supplement to the Author's 'Catechism of the Steam Engine.' By JOHN BOURNE, C.E. New Edition, including many New Examples; with 124 Woodcuts. Fcp. 8vo. 6s.

A TREATISE on the SCREW PROPELLER, SCREW VESSELS, and Screw Engines, as adapted for purposes of Peace and War; with Notices of other Methods of Propulsion, Tables of the Dimensions and Performance of Screw Steamers, and detailed Specifications of Ships and Engines. By J. BOURNE, C.E. New Edition, with 54 Plates and 287 Woodcuts. 4to. 63s.

EXAMPLES of MODERN STEAM, AIR, and GAS ENGINES of the most Approved Types, as employed for Pumping, for Driving Machinery, for Locomotion, and for Agriculture, minutely and practically described. By JOHN BOURNE, C.E. In course of publication in 24 Parts, price 2s. 6d. each, forming One volume 4to. with about 50 Plates and 400 Woodcuts.

A HISTORY of the MACHINE-WROUGHT HOSIERY and LACE Manufactures. By WILLIAM FELKIN, F.L.S. F.S.S. Royal 8vo. 21s.

PRACTICAL TREATISE on METALLURGY, adapted from the last German Edition of Professor KERL'S *Metallurgy* by W. CROOKES, F.R.S. &c. and E. RÖHRIG, Ph.D. M.E. With 625 Woodcuts. 3 vols. 8vo. price £4 19s.

MITCHELL'S MANUAL of PRACTICAL ASSAYING. Third Edition, for the most part re-written, with all the recent Discoveries incorporated, by W. CROOKES, F.R.S. With 188 Woodcuts. 8vo. 28s.

The ART of PERFUMERY; the History and Theory of Odours, and the Methods of Extracting the Aromas of Plants. By Dr. PIESSE, F.C.S. Third Edition, with 53 Woodcuts. Crown 8vo. 10s. 6d.

LOUDON'S ENCYCLOPÆDIA of AGRICULTURE: comprising the Laying-out, Improvement, and Management of Landed Property, and the Cultivation and Economy of the Productions of Agriculture. With 1,100 Woodcuts. 8vo. 21s.

Loudon's Encyclopædia of Gardening: comprising the Theory and Practice of Horticulture, Floriculture, Arboriculture, and Landscape Gardening. With 1,000 Woodcuts. 8vo. 21s.

BAYLDON'S ART of VALUING RENTS and TILLAGES, and Claims of Tenants upon Quitting Farms, both at Michaelmas and Lady-Day. Eighth Edition, revised by J. C. MORTON. 8vo. 10s. 6d.

Religious and *Moral Works.*

AUTHORITY and CONSCIENCE; a Free Debate on the Tendency of Dogmatic Theology and on the Characteristics of Faith. Edited by CONWAY MOREL. Post 8vo. price 7s. 6d.

REASONS of FAITH; or, the ORDER of the Christian Argument Developed and Explained. By the Rev. G. S. DREW, M.A. Second Edition, revised and enlarged. Fcp. 8vo. price 6s.

CHRIST the CONSOLER; a Book of Comfort for the Sick. With a Preface by the Right Rev. the Lord Bishop of Carlisle. Small 8vo. price 6s.

The TRUE DOCTRINE of the EUCHARIST. By THOMAS S. L. VOGAN, D.D. Canon and Prebendary of Chichester and Rural Dean. 8vo. price 18s.

CHRISTIAN SACERDOTALISM, viewed from a Layman's standpoint or tried by Holy Scripture and the Early Fathers ; with a short Sketch of the State of the Church from the end of the Third to the Reformation in the beginning of the Sixteenth Century. By JOHN JARDINE, M.A. LL.D. 8vo. price 8s. 6d.

SYNONYMS of the OLD TESTAMENT, their BEARING on CHRISTIAN FAITH and PRACTICE. By the Rev. ROBERT BAKER GIRDLESTONE, M.A. 8vo. price 15s.

An INTRODUCTION to the THEOLOGY of the CHURCH of ENGLAND, in an Exposition of the Thirty-nine Articles. By the Rev. T. P. BOULTBEE, LL.D. Fcp. 8vo. price 6s.

FUNDAMENTALS; or, Bases of Belief concerning MAN and GOD: a Handbook of Mental, Moral, and Religious Philosophy. By the Rev. T. GRIFFITH, M.A. 8vo. price 10s. 6d.

PRAYERS SELECTED from the COLLECTION of the late BARON BUNSEN, and Translated by CATHERINE WINKWORTH. PART I. For the Family. PART II. Prayers and Meditations for Private Use. Fcp. 8vo. price 3s. 6d.

The STUDENT'S COMPENDIUM of the BOOK of COMMON PRAYER; being Notes Historical and Explanatory of the Liturgy of the Church of England. By the Rev. H. ALLDEN NASH. Fcp. 8vo. price 2s. 6d.

The TRUTH of the BIBLE: Evidence from the Mosaic and other Records of Creation; the Origin and Antiquity of Man; the Science of Scripture; and from the Archæology of Different Nations of the Earth. By the Rev. B. W. SAVILE, M.A. Crown 8vo. price 7s. 6d.

CHURCHES and their CREEDS. By the Rev. Sir PHILIP PERRING, Bart. late Scholar of Trin. Coll. Cambridge, and University Medallist. Crown 8vo. price 10s. 6d.

CONSIDERATIONS on the REVISION of the ENGLISH NEW TESTAMENT. By C. J. ELLICOTT, D.D. Lord Bishop of Gloucester and Bristol. Post 8vo. price 5s. 6d.

An EXPOSITION of the 39 ARTICLES, Historical and Doctrinal. By E. HAROLD BROWNE, D.D. Lord Bishop of Ely. Ninth Edit. 8vo. 16s.,

The **LIFE** and **EPISTLES** of **ST. PAUL.** By the Rev. W. J.
CONYBEARE, M.A., and the Very Rev. J. S. HOWSON, D.D. Dean of Chester:—
LIBRARY EDITION, with all the Original Illustrations, Maps, Landscapes
on Steel, Woodcuts, &c. 2 vols. 4to. 48s.
INTERMEDIATE EDITION, with a Selection of Maps, Plates, and Woodcuts.
2 vols. square crown 8vo. 31s. 6d.
STUDENT'S EDITION, revised and condensed, with 46 Illustrations and
Maps. 1 vol. crown 8vo. price 9s.

The **VOYAGE** and **SHIPWRECK** of **ST. PAUL;** with Dissertations
on the Life and Writings of St. Luke and the Ships and Navigation of the
Ancients. By JAMES SMITH, F.R.S. Third Edition. Crown 8vo. 10s. 6d.

A CRITICAL and **GRAMMATICAL COMMENTARY** on **ST. PAUL'S**
Epistles. By C. J. ELLICOTT, D.D. Lord Bishop of Gloucester & Bristol. 8vo.

Galatians, Fourth Edition, 8s. 6d.

Ephesians, Fourth Edition, 8s. 6d.

Pastoral Epistles, Fourth Edition, 10s. 6d.

Philippians, Colossians, and **Philemon,** Third Edition, 10s. 6d.

Thessalonians, Third Edition, 7s. 6d.

HISTORICAL LECTURES on the **LIFE** of **OUR LORD JESUS**
CHRIST: being the Hulsean Lectures for 1859. By C. J. ELLICOTT, D.D.
Lord Bishop of Gloucester and Bristol. Fifth Edition. 8vo. price 12s.

EVIDENCE of the **TRUTH** of the **CHRISTIAN RELIGION** derived
from the Literal Fulfilment of Prophecy. By ALEXANDER KEITH, D.D.
37th Edition, with numerous Plates, in square 8vo. 12s. 6d.; also the 39th
Edition, in post 8vo. with 5 Plates, 6s.

History and **Destiny** of the **World** and **Church,** according to
Scripture. By the same Author. Square 8vo. with 40 Illustrations, 10s.

An **INTRODUCTION** to the **STUDY** of the **NEW TESTAMENT,**
Critical, Exegetical, and Theological. By the Rev. S. DAVIDSON, D.D.
LL.D. 2 vols. 8vo. 30s.

HARTWELL HORNE'S INTRODUCTION to the **CRITICAL STUDY**
and Knowledge of the Holy Scriptures, as last revised; with 4 Maps and
22 Woodcuts and Facsimiles. 4 vols. 8vo. 42s.

EWALD'S HISTORY of **ISRAEL** to the **DEATH** of **MOSES.** Translated from the German. Edited, with a Preface and an Appendix, by RUSSELL
MARTINEAU, M.A. Second Edition. 2 vols. 8vo. 24s. VOLS. III. and IV.
edited by J. E. CARPENTER, M.A. price 21s.

The **HISTORY** and **LITERATURE** of the **ISRAELITES,** according
to the Old Testament and the Apocrypha. By C. DE ROTHSCHILD and
A. DE ROTHSCHILD. Second Edition, revised. 2 vols. post 8vo. with Two
Maps, price 12s. 6d. Abridged Edition, in 1 vol. fcp. 8vo. price 3s. 6d.

The **SEE** of **ROME** in the **MIDDLE AGES.** By the Rev. OSWALD
J. REICHEL, B.C.L. and M.A. 8vo. price 18s.

The **TREASURY** of **BIBLE KNOWLEDGE;** being a Dictionary of the
Books, Persons, Places, Events, and other matters of which mention is made
in Holy Scripture. By Rev. J. AYRE, M.A. With Maps, 16 Plates, and
numerous Woodcuts. Fcp. 8vo. price 6s. cloth, or 9s. 6d. neatly bound in calf.

The GREEK TESTAMENT; with Notes, Grammatical and Exegetical. By the Rev. W. WEBSTER, M.A. and the Rev. W. F. WILKINSON, M.A. 2 vols. 8vo. £2 4s.

EVERY-DAY SCRIPTURE DIFFICULTIES explained and illustrated. By J. E. PRESCOTT, M.A. VOL. I. *Matthew* and *Mark*; VOL. II. *Luke* and *John*. 2 vols. 8vo. 9s. each.

The PENTATEUCH and BOOK of JOSHUA CRITICALLY EXAMINED. By the Right Rev. J. W. COLENSO, D.D. Lord Bishop of Natal. People's Edition, in 1 vol. crown 8vo. 6s.

PART VI. *the Later Legislation of the Pentateuch.* 8vo. price 24s.

The FORMATION of CHRISTENDOM. By T. W. ALLIES. PARTS I. and II. 8vo. price 12s. each Part.

ENGLAND and CHRISTENDOM. By ARCHBISHOP MANNING, D.D. Post 8vo. price 10s. 6d.

A VIEW of the SCRIPTURE REVELATIONS CONCERNING a FUTURE STATE. By RICHARD WHATELY, D.D. late Archbishop of Dublin. Ninth Edition. Fcp. 8vo. 5s.¦

THOUGHTS for the AGE. By ELIZABETH M. SEWELL, Author of 'Amy Herbert' &c. New Edition, revised. Fcp. 8vo. price 5s.

Passing Thoughts on Religion. By the same Author. Fcp. 8vo. 3s. 6d.

Self-Examination before Confirmation. By the same Author. 32mo. price 1s. 6d.

Readings for a Month Preparatory to Confirmation, from Writers of the Early and English Church. By the same Author. Fcp. 4s.

Readings for Every Day in Lent, compiled from the Writings of Bishop JEREMY TAYLOR. By the same Author. Fcp. 5s.

Preparation for the Holy Communion; the Devotions chiefly from the works of JEREMY TAYLOR. By the same Author. 32mo. 3s.

THOUGHTS for the HOLY WEEK for Young Persons. By the Author of 'Amy Herbert.' New Edition. Fcp. 8vo. 2s.

PRINCIPLES of EDUCATION Drawn from Nature and Revelation, and applied to Female Education in the Upper Classes. By the Author of 'Amy Herbert.' 2 vols. fcp. 12s. 6d.

SINGERS and SONGS of the CHURCH: being Biographical Sketches of the Hymn-Writers in all the principal Collections; with Notes on their Psalms and Hymns. By JOSIAH MILLER, M.A. Post 8vo. price 10s. 6d.

LYRA GERMANICA, translated from the German by Miss C. WINKWORTH. FIRST SERIES, Hymns for the Sundays and Chief Festivals. SECOND SERIES, the Christian Life. Fcp. 3s. 6d. each SERIES.

'SPIRITUAL SONGS' for the SUNDAYS and HOLIDAYS throughout the Year. By J. S. B. MONSELL, LL.D. Vicar of Egham and Rural Dean. Fourth Edition, Sixth Thousand. Fcp. 4s. 6d.

The BEATITUDES: Abasement before God; Sorrow for Sin; Meekness of Spirit; Desire for Holiness; Gentleness; Purity of Heart; the Peacemakers; Sufferings for Christ. By the same. Third Edition. Fcp. 3s. 6d.

His PRESENCE—not his MEMORY, 1855. By the same Author, in Memory of his SON. Sixth Edition. 16mo. 1s.

ENDEAVOURS after the CHRISTIAN LIFE: Discourses. By JAMES MARTINEAU. Fourth Edition, carefully revised. Post 8vo. 7s. 6d.

WHATELY'S INTRODUCTORY LESSONS on the CHRISTIAN Evidences. 18mo. 6d.

FOUR DISCOURSES of CHRYSOSTOM, chiefly on the Parable of the Rich Man and Lazarus. Translated by F. ALLEN, B.A. Crown 8vo. 3s. 6d.

BISHOP JEREMY TAYLOR'S ENTIRE WORKS. With Life by BISHOP HEBER. Revised and corrected by the Rev. C. P. EDEN, 10 vols. price £5 5s.

Travels, Voyages, &c.

HOW to SEE NORWAY. By Captain J. R. CAMPBELL. With Map and 5 Woodcuts. Fcp. 8vo. price 5s.

PAU and the PYRENEES. By Count HENRY RUSSELL, Member of the Alpine Club, &c. With 2 Maps. Fcp. 8vo. price 5s.

SCENES in the SUNNY SOUTH; including the Atlas Mountains and the Oases of the Sahara in Algeria. By Lieut.-Col. the Hon. C. S. VEREKER, M.A. Commandant of the Limerick Artillery Militia. 2 vols. post 8vo. price 21s.

The **PLAYGROUND of EUROPE.** By LESLIE STEPHEN, late President of the Alpine Club. With 4 Illustrations engraved on Wood by E. Whymper. Crown 8vo. price 10s. 6d.

CADORE; or, TITIAN'S COUNTRY. By JOSIAH GILBERT, one of the Authors of 'The Dolomite Mountains.' With Map, Facsimile, and 40 Illustrations. Imperial 8vo. 31s. 6d.

HOURS of EXERCISE in the ALPS. By JOHN TYNDALL, LL.D. F.R.S. Second Edition, with 7 Woodcuts by E. WHYMPER. Crown 8vo. price 12s. 6d.

TRAVELS in the CENTRAL CAUCASUS and BASHAN. Including Visits to Ararat and Tabreez and Ascents of Kazbek and Elbruz. By D. W. FRESHFIELD. Square crown 8vo. with Maps, &c. 18s.

PICTURES in TYROL and Elsewhere. From a Family Sketch-Book. By the Authoress of 'A Voyage en Zigzag,' &c. Second Edition. Small 4to. with numerous Illustrations, 21s.

HOW WE SPENT the SUMMER; or, a Voyage en Zigzag in Switzer-land and Tyrol with some Members of the ALPINE CLUB. From the Sketch-Book of one of the Party. In oblong 4to. with 300 Illustrations, 15s.

BEATEN TRACKS; or, Pen and Pencil Sketches in Italy. By the Authoress of 'A Voyage en Zigzag.' With 42 Plates, containing about 200 Sketches from Drawings made on the Spot. 8vo. 16s.

MAP of the CHAIN of MONT BLANC, from an actual Survey in 1863—1864. By A. ADAMS-REILLY, F.R.G.S. M.A.C. Published under the Authority of the Alpine Club. In Chromolithography on extra stout drawing-paper 28in. × 17in. price 10s. or mounted on canvas in a folding case, 12s. 6d.

WESTWARD by RAIL; the New Route to the East. By W. F. RAE. With Map shewing the Lines of Rail between the Atlantic and the Pacific and Sections of the Railway. Second Edition. Post 8vo. price 10s. 6d.

HISTORY of DISCOVERY in our AUSTRALASIAN COLONIES, Australia, Tasmania, and New Zealand, from the Earliest Date to the Present Day. By WILLIAM HOWITT. 2 vols. 8vo. with 3 Maps, 20s.

ZIGZAGGING AMONGST DOLOMITES. By the Author of 'How we Spent the Summer, or a Voyage en Zigzag in Switzerland and Tyrol.' With upwards of 300 Illustrations by the Author. Oblong 4to. price 15s.

The DOLOMITE MOUNTAINS; Excursions through Tyrol, Carinthia, Carniola, and Friuli, 1861-1863. By J. GILBERT and G. C. CHURCHILL, F.R.G.S. With numerous Illustrations. Square crown 8vo. 21s.

GUIDE to the PYRENEES, for the use of Mountaineers. By CHARLES PACKE. 2nd Edition, with Map and Illustrations. Cr. 8vo. 7s. 6d.

The ALPINE GUIDE. By JOHN BALL, M.R.I.A. late President of the Alpine Club. Thoroughly Revised Editions, in Three Volumes, post 8vo. with Maps and other Illustrations:—

GUIDE to the WESTERN ALPS, including Mont Blanc, Monte Rosa, Zermatt, &c. Price 6s. 6d.

GUIDE to the CENTRAL ALPS, including all the Oberland District. Price 7s. 6d.

GUIDE to the EASTERN ALPS, price 10s. 6d.

Introduction on Alpine Travelling in General, and on the Geology of the Alps, price 1s. Each of the Three Volumes or Parts of the *Alpine Guide* may be had with this INTRODUCTION prefixed, price 1s. extra.

VISITS to REMARKABLE PLACES: Old Halls, Battle-Fields, and Stones Illustrative of Striking Passages in English History and Poetry. By WILLIAM HOWITT. 2 vols. square crown 8vo. with Woodcuts, 25s.

The RURAL LIFE of ENGLAND. By the same Author. With Woodcuts by Bewick and Williams. Medium 8vo. 12s. 6d.

Works of *Fiction.*

POPULAR ROMANCES of the MIDDLE AGES. By GEORGE W. COX, M.A. Author of 'The Mythology of the Aryan Nations' &c. and EUSTACE HINTON JONES. Crown 8vo. price 10s. 6d.

HARTLAND FOREST; a Legend of North Devon. By Mrs. BRAY, Author of 'The White Hoods,' 'Life of Stothard,' &c. Post 8vo. with Frontispiece, price 4s. 6d.

NOVELS and TALES. By the Right Hon. B. DISRAELI, M.P. Cabinet Edition, complete in Ten Volumes, crown 8vo. price 6s. each, as follows:—

LOTHAIR, 6s.
CONINGSBY, 6s.
SYBIL, 6s.
TANCRED, 6s.
VENETIA, 6s.

HENRIETTA TEMPLE, 6s.
CONTARINI FLEMING, &c. 6s.
ALROY, IXION, &c. 6s.
The YOUNG DUKE, &c. 6s.
VIVIAN GREY, 6s.

The MODERN NOVELIST'S LIBRARY. Each Work, in crown 8vo. complete in a Single Volume:—

MELVILLE'S GLADIATORS, 2s. boards; 2s. 6d. cloth.
———————— GOOD FOR NOTHING, 2s. boards; 2s. 6d. cloth.
———————— HOLMBY HOUSE, 2s. boards; 2s. 6d. cloth.
———————— INTERPRETER, 2s. boards; 2s. 6d. cloth.
———————— KATE COVENTRY, 2s. boards; 2s. 6d. cloth.
———————— QUEEN'S MARIES, 2s. boards; 2s. 6d. cloth.
TROLLOPE'S WARDEN, 1s. 6d. boards; 2s. cloth.
———————— BARCHESTER TOWERS, 2s. boards; 2s. 6d. cloth.
BRAMLEY-MOORE'S SIX SISTERS of the VALLEYS, 2s. boards; 2s. 6d. cloth.

IERNE; a Tale. By W. STEUART TRENCH, Author of 'Realities of Irish Life.' Second Edition. 2 vols. post 8vo. price 21s.

The HOME at HEATHERBRAE; a Tale. By the Author of 'Everley.' Fcp. 8vo. price 5s.

CABINET EDITION of STORIES and TALES by MISS SEWELL:—

AMY HERBERT, 2s.6d.
GERTRUDE, 2s. 6d.
The EARL'S DAUGHTER, 2s. 6d.
EXPERIENCE of LIFE, 2s. 6d.
CLEVE HALL, 3s. 6d.

IVORS, 3s. 6d.
KATHARINE ASHTON, 3s. 6d.
MARGARET PERCIVAL, 5s.
LANETON PARSONAGE, 3s. 6d.
URSULA, 4s. 6d.

STORIES and TALES. By E. M. SEWELL. Comprising:—Amy Herbert; Gertrude; The Earl's Daughter; The Experience of Life; Cleve Hall; Ivors; Katharine Ashton; Margaret Percival; Laneton Parsonage; and Ursula. The Ten Works, complete in Eight Volumes, crown 8vo. bound in leather, and contained in a Box, price 42s.

A Glimpse of the World. By the Author of 'Amy Herbert.' Fcp. 7s. 6d.

The Journal of a Home Life. By the same Author. Post 8vo. 9s. 6d.

After Life; a Sequel to 'The Journal of a Home Life.' Price 10s. 6d.

UNCLE PETER'S FAIRY TALE for the NINETEENTH CENTURY. Edited by E. M. SEWELL, Author of 'Amy Herbert,' &c. Fcp. 8vo. 7s. 6d.

THE GIANT; A Witch's Story for English Boys. By the same Author and Editor. Fcp. 8vo. price 5s.

WONDERFUL STORIES from NORWAY, SWEDEN, and ICELAND. Adapted and arranged by JULIA GODDARD. With an Introductory Essay by the Rev. G. W. COX, M.A. and Six Woodcuts. Square post 8vo. 6s.

A VISIT to MY DISCONTENTED COUSIN. Reprinted, with some Additions, from Fraser's Magazine. Crown 8vo. price 7s. 6d.

BECKER'S GALLUS; or, Roman Scenes of the Time of Augustus: with Notes and Excursuses. New Edition. Post 8vo. 7s. 6d.

BECKER'S CHARICLES; a Tale illustrative of Private Life among the Ancient Greeks: with Notes and Excursuses. New Edition. Post 8vo. 7s. 6d.

CABINET EDITION of NOVELS and TALES by G. J. WHYTE
MELVILLE :—

DIGBY GRAND, 5s.

KATE COVENTRY, 5s.

GENERAL BOUNCE, 5s.

HOLMBY HOUSE, 5s.

The QUEEN'S MARIES, 6s.

The INTERPRETER, 5s.

GOOD FOR NOTHING, price 6s.

TALES of ANCIENT GREECE. By GEORGE W. COX, M.A. late Scholar of Trin. Coll. Oxon. Crown 8vo. price 6s. 6d.

A MANUAL of MYTHOLOGY, in the form of Question and Answer. By the same Author. Fcp. 3s.

OUR CHILDREN'S STORY, by one of their Gossips. By the Author of 'Voyage en Zigzag,' 'Pictures in Tyrol,' &c. Small 4to. with Sixty Illustrations by the Author, price 10s. 6d.

Poetry and The Drama.

A VISION of CREATION, a POEM; with an Introduction, Geological and Critical. By CUTHBERT COLLINGWOOD, M.A. and B.M. Oxon. F.L.S. &c. Author of 'Rambles of a Naturalist on the Shores and Waters of the China Seas,' &c. Crown 8vo. price 7s. 6d.

The STORY of GAUTAMA BUDDHA and his CREED; an Epic. By RICHARD PHILLIPS. Squara fcp. 8vo. price 6s.

BALLADS and LYRICS of OLD FRANCE; with other Poems. By A. LANG, Fellow of Merton College, Oxford. Square fcp. 8vo. price 5s.

SONGS of the SIERRAS. By JOAQUIN MILLER. New Edition, revised by the Author. Fcp. 8vo. price 6s.

THOMAS MOORE'S POETICAL WORKS, with the Author's last Copyright Additions :—

SHAMROCK EDITION, crown 8vo. price 3s. 6d.

PEOPLE'S EDITION, square crown 8vo. with Illustrations, price 10s. 6d.

LIBRARY EDITION, medium 8vo. Portrait and Vignette, 14s.

MOORE'S IRISH MELODIES, Maclise's Edition, with 161 Steel Plates from Original Drawings. Super-royal 8vo. 31s. 6d.

Miniature Edition of Moore's Irish Melodies with Maclise's Designs (as above) reduced in Lithography. Imp. 16mo. 10s. 6d.

MOORE'S LALLA ROOKH. Tenniel's Edition, with 68 Wood Engravings from original Drawings and other Illustrations. Fcp. 4to. 21s.

SOUTHEY'S POETICAL WORKS, with the Author's last Corrections and copyright Additions. Library Edition, in 1 vol. medium 8vo. with Portrait and Vignette, 14s.

LAYS of ANCIENT ROME; with Ivry and the Armada. By the Right Hon. LORD MACAULAY. 16mo. 4s. 6d.

Lord Macaulay's Lays of Ancient Rome. With 90 Illustrations on Wood, from the Antique, from Drawings by G. SCHARF. Fcp. 4to. 21s.

Miniature Edition of Lord Macaulay's Lays of Ancient Rome, with the Illustrations (as above) reduced in Lithography. Imp. 16mo. 10s. 6d.

GOLDSMITH'S POETICAL WORKS, with Wood Engravings from Designs by Members of the ETCHING CLUB. Imperial 16mo. 7s. 6d.

POEMS OF BYGONE YEARS. Edited by the Author of 'Amy Herbert' &c. Fcp. 8vo. price 5s.

The ÆNEID of VIRGIL Translated into English Verse. By JOHN CONINGTON, M.A. New Edition. Crown 8vo. 9s.

HORATII OPERA. Library Edition, with Marginal References and English Notes. Edited by the Rev. J. E. YONGE. 8vo. 21s.

BOWDLER'S FAMILY SHAKSPEARE, cheaper Genuine Editions. Medium 8vo. large type, with 36 WOODCUTS, price 14s. Cabinet Edition, with the same ILLUSTRATIONS, 6 vols. fcp. 3s. 6d. each.

POEMS. By JEAN INGELOW. Fifteenth Edition. Fcp. 8vo. 5s.

POEMS by Jean Ingelow. With nearly 100 Illustrations by Eminent Artists, engraved on Wood by the Brothers DALZIEL. Fcp. 4to. 21s.

A STORY of DOOM, and other Poems. By JEAN INGELOW. Third Edition. Fcp. 5s.

JOHN JERNINGHAM'S JOURNAL. Fcp. 8vo. price 3s. 6d.

The MAD WAR PLANET, and other **POEMS.** By WILLIAM HOWITT, Author of 'Visits to Remarkable Places' &c. Fcp. 8vo. price 5s.

EUCHARIS; a Poem. By F. REGINALD STATHAM (Francis Reynolds), Author of 'Alice Rushton, and other Poems' and 'Glaphyra, and other Poems.' Fcp. 8vo. price 3s. 6d.

WORKS by EDWARD YARDLEY:—
    FANTASTIC STORIES. Fcp. 3s. 6d.
    MELUSINE *and* OTHER POEMS. Fcp. 5s.
    HORACE'S ODES, *translated into* English Verse. Crown 8vo. 6s.
    SUPPLEMENTARY STORIES *and* POEMS. Fcp. 3s. 6d.

Rural Sports, &c.

ENCYCLOPÆDIA of RURAL SPORTS; a complete Account, Historical, Practical, and Descriptive, of Hunting, Shooting, Fishing, Racing, and all other Rural and Athletic Sports and Pastimes. By D. P. BLAINE. With above 600 Woodcuts (20 from Designs by JOHN LEECH). 8vo. 21s.

The DEAD SHOT, or Sportsman's Complete Guide; a Treatise on the Use of the Gun, Dog-breaking, Pigeon-shooting, &c. By MARKSMAN. Revised Edition. Fcp. 8vo. with Plates, 5s.

The FLY-FISHER'S ENTOMOLOGY. By ALFRED RONALDS. With coloured Representations of the Natural and Artificial Insect. Sixth Edition; with 20 coloured Plates. 8vo. 14s.

A BOOK on ANGLING; a complete Treatise on the Art of Angling in every branch. By FRANCIS FRANCIS. New Edition, with Portrait and 15 other Plates, plain and coloured. Post 8vo. 15s.

The BOOK of the ROACH. By GREVILLE FENNELL, of ' The Field.' Fcp. 8vo. price 2s. 6d.

WILCOCKS'S SEA-FISHERMAN; comprising the Chief Methods of Hook and Line Fishing in the British and other Seas, a Glance at Nets, and Remarks on Boats and Boating. Second Edition, enlarged; with 80 Woodcuts. Post 8vo. 12s. 6d.

HORSES and STABLES. By Colonel F. FITZWYGRAM, XV. the King's Hussars. With Twenty-four Plates of Illustrations, containing very numerous Figures engraved on Wood. 8vo. 15s.

The HORSE'S FOOT, and HOW to KEEP IT SOUND. By W. MILES, Esq. Ninth Edition, with Illustrations. Imperial 8vo. 12s. 6d.

A PLAIN TREATISE on HORSE-SHOEING. By the same Author. Sixth Edition. Post 8vo. with Illustrations, 2s. 6d.

STABLES and STABLE-FITTINGS. By the same. Imp. 8vo. with 13 Plates, 15s.

REMARKS on HORSES' TEETH, addressed to Purchasers. By the same. Post 8vo. 1s. 6d.

A TREATISE on HORSE-SHOEING and LAMENESS. By JOSEPH GAMGEE, Veterinary Surgeon, formerly Lecturer on the Principles and Practice of Farriery in the New Veterinary College, Edinburgh. 8vo. with 55 Woodcuts, price 15s.

BLAINE'S VETERINARY ART; a Treatise on the Anatomy, Physiology, and Curative Treatment of the Diseases of the Horse, Neat Cattle and Sheep. Seventh Edition, revised and enlarged by C. STEEL, M.R.C.V.S.L. 8vo. with Plates and Woodcuts, 18s.

The HORSE: with a Treatise on Draught. By WILLIAM YOUATT. New Edition, revised and enlarged. 8vo. with numerous Woodcuts, 12s. 6d.

The DOG. By the same Author. 8vo. with numerous Woods, 6s.

The DOG in HEALTH and DISEASE. By STONEHENGE. With 70 Wood Engravings. Square crown 8vo. 10s. 6d.

The GREYHOUND. By STONEHENGE. Revised Edition, with 24 Portraits of Greyhounds. Square crown 8vo. 10s. 6d.

The OX; his Diseases and their Treatment: with an Essay on Parturition in the Cow. By J. R. DOBSON. Crown 8vo. with Illustrations, 7s. 6d.

Works of Utility and General Information.

The THEORY and PRACTICE of BANKING. By H. D. MACLEOD, M.A. Barrister-at-Law. Second Edition, entirely remodelled. 2 vols. 8vo. 30s.

A DICTIONARY, Practical, Theoretical, and Historical, of Commerce and Commercial Navigation. By J. R. M'CULLOCH. New and thoroughly revised Edition. 8vo. price 63s. cloth, or 70s. half-bd. in russia.

The LAW of NATIONS Considered as Independent Political Communities. By Sir TRAVERS TWISS, D.C.L. 2 vols. 8vo. 30s.; or separately, PART I. Peace, 12s. PART II. War, 18s.

The CABINET LAWYER ; a Popular Digest of the Laws of England, Civil, Criminal, and Constitutional: intended for Practical Use and General Information. Twenty-third Edition. Fcp. 8vo. price 7s. 6d.

PEWTNER'S COMPREHENSIVE SPECIFIER ; a Guide to the Practical Specification of every kind of Building-Artificers' Work; with Forms of Building Conditions and Agreements, an Appendix, Foot-Notes, and a copious Index. Edited by W. YOUNG, Architect. Crown 8vo. price 6s.

COLLIERIES and COLLIERS ; a Handbook of the Law and Leading Cases relating thereto. By J. C. FOWLER, of the Inner Temple, Barrister. Second Edition. Fcp. 8vo. 7s. 6d.

The MATERNAL MANAGEMENT of CHILDREN in HEALTH and Disease. By THOMAS BULL, M.D. Fcp. 5s.

HINTS to MOTHERS on the MANAGEMENT of their HEALTH during the Period of Pregnancy and in the Lying-in Room. By the late THOMAS BULL, M.D. Fcp. 5s.

HOW to NURSE SICK CHILDREN; containing Directions which may be found of service to all who have charge of the Young. By CHARLES WEST, M.D. Second Edition. Fcp. 8vo. 1s. 6d.

NOTES on LYING-IN INSTITUTIONS; with a Proposal for Organising an Institution for Training Midwives and Midwifery Nurses. By FLORENCE NIGHTINGALE. With 5 Plans. Square crown 8vo. 7s. 6d.

NOTES on HOSPITALS. By FLORENCE NIGHTINGALE. Third Edition, enlarged ; with 13 Plans. Post 4to. 18s.

CHESS OPENINGS. By F. W. LONGMAN, Balliol College, Oxford. Fcp. 8vo. 2s. 6d.

A PRACTICAL TREATISE on BREWING ; with Formulæ for Public Brewers, and Instructions for Private Families. By W. BLACK. 8vo. 10s. 6d.

MODERN COOKERY for PRIVATE FAMILIES, reduced to a System of Easy Practice in a Series of carefully-tested Receipts. By ELIZA ACTON. Newly revised and enlarged Edition; with 8 Plates of Figures and 150 Woodcuts. Fcp. 6s.

WILLICH'S POPULAR TABLES, for ascertaining, according to the Carlisle Table of Mortality, the value of Lifehold, Leasehold, and Church Property, Renewal Fines, Reversions, &c. Seventh Edition, edited by MONTAGUE MARRIOTT, Barrister-at-Law. Post 8vo. price 10s.

MAUNDER'S TREASURY of KNOWLEDGE and LIBRARY of Reference: comprising an English Dictionary and Grammar, Universal Gazetteer, Classical Dictionary, Chronology, Law Dictionary, a Synopsis of the Peerage, useful Tables, &c. Revised Edition. Fcp. 8vo. price 6s.

INDEX.

Spottiswoode & Co., Printers, New-street Square, London.

www.ingramcontent.com/pod-product-compliance
Lightning Source LLC
Chambersburg PA
CBHW021106270326
41929CB00009B/753